The
Mediterranean
Diet Plan

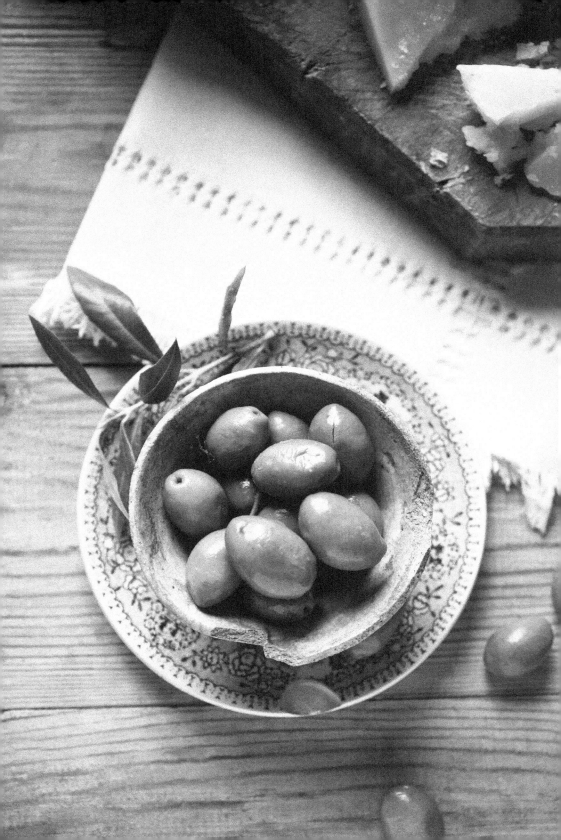

The
Mediterranean
Diet Plan

Heart-Healthy
Recipes & Meal Plans
for Every Type of Eater

SUSAN ZOGHEIB, MHS, RD, LDN

Foreword by
Phillip R. Anderson III, MD

ROCKRIDGE
PRESS

This is for you, Bibi.
Thank you for inspiring me.

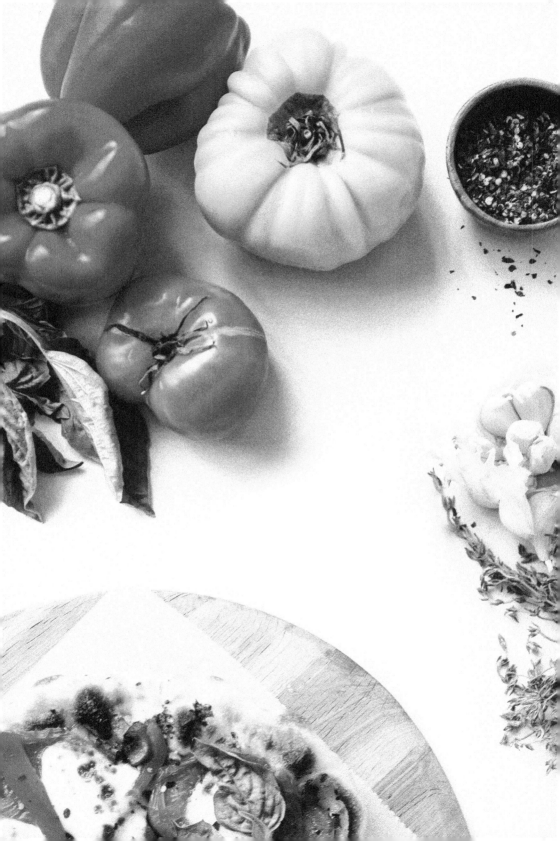

CONTENTS

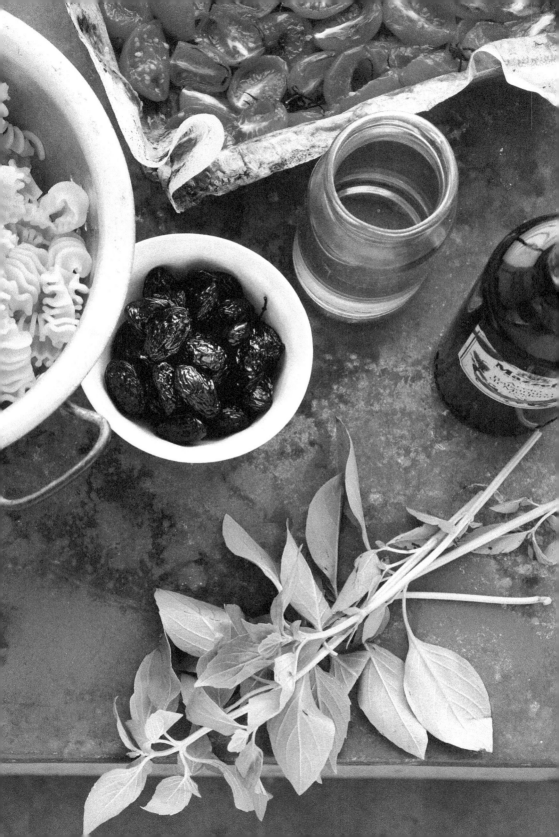

FOREWORD

The leading cause of mortality in the United States and Western civilization lies predominantly in atherosclerosis, or the development of blocked arteries of the heart. When it comes to preventing this potentially deadly disease, diet and physical activity play a huge part. From extensive research, the American Heart Association guidelines exclusively recommend the Mediterranean diet.

As a practicing clinical cardiologist, I am constantly encouraging my patients to adopt this diet. Unfortunately, many people have a negative association with the word *diet*. A healthy diet is perceived to limit the pleasure of eating—but I can't stress enough the joy of the Mediterranean diet. It encourages needed lifestyle changes to stay active and to enjoy time with family and friends— all while adopting heart-healthy foods, wine included.

Originally from the Mediterranean region, Susan is a clinical expert in nutrition and comes from a family with a long tradition in cooking. In *The Mediterranean Diet Plan*, she explains the science behind why the diet decreases cardiovascular risk and provides you with 100 delicious recipes and meal plans to begin your journey to lifelong healthy eating habits.

This book is an accessible, practical and informational tool that makes heart-healthy eating decisions a cinch. I'm thankful to have this cookbook to share with patients to help them improve their lives.

Phillip R. Anderson III, MD

Clinical Interventional Cardiologist
Codirector Florida Hospital Orlando Cardiac Rehab
CENTRAL FLORIDA CARDIOLOGY GROUP

INTRODUCTION

The Mediterranean diet developed naturally from the inhabitants, climate, and native foods of Crete, Greece's largest island. In the 1950s, Dr. Ancel Keys, from the University of Minnesota school of public health, studied seven countries and analyzed the basics of their diets in relation to the prevalence of cardiovascular diseases. It was Keys who set the foundation for what would later be called the Mediterranean diet.

The Mediterranean diet is considered one of the world's healthiest diets. The diet is associated with reduced saturated fat, which means lower levels of arterial inflammation—a risk factor for heart attack and stroke—reduced high blood pressure, a lowered risk of developing cancer, and increased prevention of life-threatening conditions. The Mediterranean diet can be easily incorporated into the daily lives of anyone looking to eat healthy and varied meals. It is abundant in fresh fruits, vegetables, whole grains, legumes, nuts, and olive oil, as well as fish, poultry, and lean sources of protein, rather than red meat. There's even a glass of red wine every day.

My experience with the Mediterranean diet started at an early age. I was born in a small remote village in the beautiful mountains of Lebanon. My aunts and uncles surrounded us. Coming from a big family, there was never a dull moment in the house. Although we lived a simple life, I had never felt so rich. Fruit trees were dispersed all around the village. Vegetables were grown in my backyard. Daily family gatherings included traditional foods around the dinner table and a mouth-watering mezza—hummus, eggplant, meat kebabs, stuffed cabbage, and tabbouleh.

Family dinners have certainly changed in the last decade as technology has advanced. Back home, we didn't have any distractions. We truly were able to enjoy each other's company without the lingering distractions of email or text messages. We genuinely savored every bite of food. Physical activity was easy—after dinner, we'd go for a walk around the village and get lost in conversation. My aunts gathered every Sunday at my grandfather's house in the village, and each brought a dish to the table. Family time, like that, is slowly diminishing. Fast food has quickly become the replacement.

Since coming to the United States and becoming a dietitian, I've seen firsthand the consequences related to poor diet and lack of physical activity. Not eating the right foods and leading a sedentary lifestyle can certainly increase your risk of developing clogged arteries, high blood pressure, and high cholesterol—all contributors to the dangers of heart disease, which is quickly becoming the leading cause of death globally, accounting for more than 17.3 million deaths per year—and it is expected to keep increasing. Heart disease now accounts for 1 in 7 deaths in the United States, killing more than 370,000 Americans each year.

Prevention plays an important role in reducing the risk of this potentially fatal disease. Research has shown that following a Mediterranean diet, in conjunction with physical activity, can reduce your risk of developing cardiovascular disease. Moreover, about 30 percent of heart attacks, strokes, and deaths from heart disease can be prevented in people at high risk if they switch to a Mediterranean diet.

If you're contemplating the benefits of the Mediterranean diet, this book is for you. With four plans to accommodate different needs and lifestyle choices, it's easy to follow. And you don't have to eat meat or seafood to enjoy the benefits of the diet. You can choose from the Traditional Mediterranean Plan, Meatless Mediterranean Plan, Seafood-Free Mediterranean Plan, or 30-Minute Mediterranean Plan. Start with the plan you feel most comfortable with and explore other plans along the way. Whichever plan you enjoy, here's to your heart health!

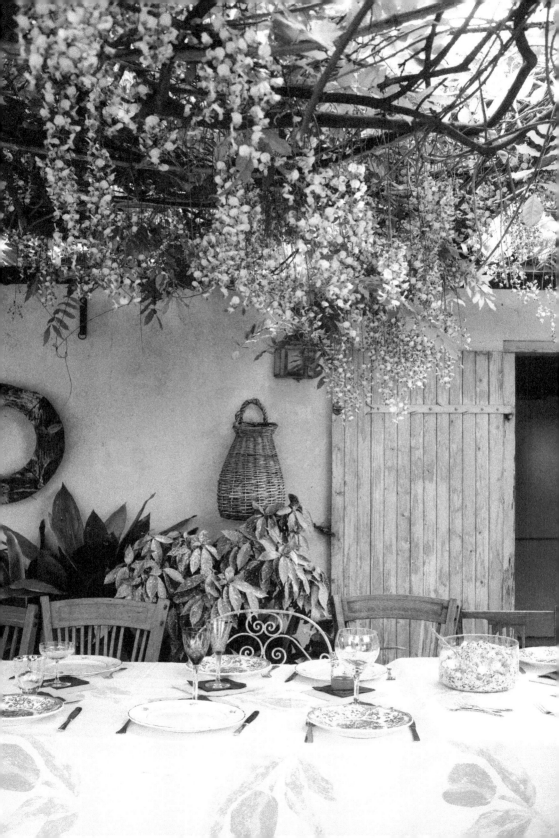

PART ONE

The Road to Better Health

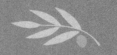

CHAPTER 1

The Mediterranean Way of Eating and Living

There's good reason for confusion whenever you open your refrigerator. From low-carb to gluten-free to paleo, the plethora of diets can be overwhelming. Despite promises to help you lose weight or improve health, rarely do diet plans meet expections and deliver results. The Mediterranean diet is an exception. It is easy to follow and understand, has been scientifically proven to improve heart health and reduce the risk of developing cancer, and doesn't require a lot of lifestyle changes. This chapter explores the history, benefits, and basics of the Mediterranean diet.

The History of the Mediterranean Diet

The Mediterranean Diet is a nutritional model originally inspired by the dietary patterns typical of the people of Crete. Through the years, the Mediterranean diet has evolved. It is closely related to the Mediterranean lifestyle and the cultural, historical, social, territorial, and environmental aspects of the people. It is not a new diet, which is precisely the reason for its strengths; in fact, its early origins even incorporated the famous Biblical seven species—wheat, barley, grapes, figs, pomegranates, olives, and date honey. These foods—along with other indigenous foods of the Middle East—are now scientifically recognized as healthy foods and have been incorporated into a heart-healthy diet.

Times have changed, though, and we don't live today like they used to in Crete. With decreased physical activity and increased calorie intake, our health is in jeopardy—and it's no surprise obesity and disease are on the rise. Fat intake has increased and fiber intake has decreased. The consumption of complex carbohydrates, fruits, and vegetables has also decreased. In the United States alone, mortality rates due to cancer and cardiovascular disease are more than three times higher than in Crete. We see meals move from the dining room to the living room in front of the television, which encourages quick meals and discourages communication and portion control. All good reasons to take a look at how we're eating and adopt healthier habits.

Discovering the Health Benefits

Over the years many diets have received attention, but the strongest evidence for beneficial health effects and decreased mortality comes from studies of the Mediterranean diet. Research has shown that the Mediterranean diet is effective at warding off cardiovascular disease and premature death, and enhancing weight loss. A 2013 study looked at dietary habits of more than

10,000 women and compared them to how the women were, health-wise, 15 years later. They found that women during middle age who followed a healthy diet, the Mediterranean diet or similar, were about 40% more likely to live past the age of 70 without chronic illness.

Reducing Your Risk of Cardiovascular Disease

The discovery of the health benefits of the Mediterranean diet is attributed to the American scientist Ancel Keys, who, for the first time, pointed out the correlation between cardiovascular disease and diet from various parts of the world. In 1950, Ancel Keys led the famous "Seven Countries Study," which was conducted in Finland, Holland, Italy, the United States, Greece, Japan, and (then) Yugoslavia to document the relationship between lifestyles, nutrition, and cardiovascular disease in different populations. The Seven Countries Study included cross-sectional studies able to scientifically prove the nutritional value of the Mediterranean diet and its contribution to health.

From this study emerged a clear relationship between the Mediterranean diet and decreased levels of both cholesterol and the prevalence of coronary heart disease. This was mainly due to the inclusion of the many fresh fruits and vegetables, olive oil, herbs, garlic, red onions, and other foods of vegetable origin, as well as a rather moderate consumption of red meat. Fresh and natural ingredients have more vitamins and minerals than processed foods. These factors resulted in a diet high in heart-healthy nutrients and low in saturated fats and added sugars.

A Longer Life

It is no coincidence that those living along the Mediterranean coast have some of the world's longest life spans. The climate ensures that fruits, vegetables, olives, beans, and fish are abundant, which are all rich in the antioxidants that can combat aging triggered by pollution and stress. They are also powerful fighters against the inflammation driving so many chronic diseases, such as heart disease and cancer.

A study at Harvard Medical School and Brigham and Women's Hospital looked at 4,676 women enrolled in the Nurses' Health Study, an ongoing trial tracking the health and habits of more than 120,000 registered nurses in the United States since 1976. Researchers found that women who ate a Mediterranean diet had cells that were different from those whose diets were heavier in saturated fats. The Mediterranean diet followers had longer telomeres, or bits of DNA located at the tips of chromosomes. Telomeres shorten every time a cell divides; they shrink by half from infancy to adulthood, and again by half among the elderly. It has been studied and shown that longer telomeres are linked to longer life spans.

Weight Loss

When the Mediterranean diet is combined with portion control and physical activity, it can help reduce body weight. A 2011 study published in the journal *Metabolic Syndrome and Related Disorders* evaluated the effect of the Mediterranean diet on body weight in randomized controlled trials using studies of the Mediterranean diet and weight loss since 2010. They found 16 randomized trials with more than 3,000 participants (1,848 assigned to a Mediterranean diet and 1,588 assigned to a control diet). In a six-month period, both groups had lost the same amount of weight, but those following the Mediterranean diet were able to keep the weight off for a longer period of time. The authors concluded that maintaining a Mediterranean diet could have a long-term positive effect on obtaining a healthy body weight, especially when calorie restricted and combined with physical activity.

Mediterranean Diet Principles

From Morocco to France to Italy to Greece to Spain to Lebanon, and beyond, the Mediterranean diet encompasses the traditional ingredients and recipes used by the 16 countries that border the Mediterranean Sea. While all of these countries have a colorful diet consisting of the fundamental ingredients we consider part of the Mediterranean plan, naturally, some of the cultures, religions, and lifestyles of people living in these countries vary substantially, depending on their economy and agriculture.

A hallmark of Mediterranean dishes is the simple, delicious, and natural ingredients found throughout the coastal region of the Mediterranean. With a variety of fruits and vegetables, healthy fats, whole grains, beans, poultry, beef, fish, and red wine, it's no wonder the Mediterranean diet is considered one of the healthiest diets. Luckily, you don't have to travel to Greece to adopt the Mediterranean diet. Here are the basic principles and foods usually eaten on this diet:

> *More fruits and vegetables.* Fresh fruits and vegetables are an integral part of the Mediterranean diet. Many are low in fat and high in fiber, making them heart healthy and important for weight loss. There are also a lot of antioxidants in fruits and vegetables, which reduce inflammation in our cells and help slow the aging process. Antioxidants include vitamins A, C, E, and K, which also help remove harmful free radicals— molecules that can cause oxidation of LDL, or bad cholesterol, which can clog arteries.

> *Increased whole grains.* The Mediterranean diet incorporates whole grains. Unlike refined grains that have been stripped of nutrients, whole grains are better and more nutritious for you. Whole grains contain the germ, endosperm, and bran, in contrast to refined grains, which retain only the endosperm and are made of processed ingredients. Some whole grains are barley, brown rice, bulgur, millet, oat, rye, teff, and wheat. Whole grains have several benefits, including satiety, and they contain good amounts of nutrients and naturally occurring disease-fighting chemicals called phytochemicals.

> *Drizzle some olive oil.* The Mediterranean diet's secrets lie in its use of olive oil and its style of cooking. Instead of butter, most meals are prepared with olive oil. It is used liberally in many dishes and is also poured onto salads and mixed with pasta dishes. Olive oil is packed with monounsaturated fats; it offers protection against heart disease because it keeps

LDL (bad) cholesterol levels low while increasing HDL (good) cholesterol levels. And rather than frying foods, many foods included in the Mediterranean diet are grilled or baked. These cooking methods also reduce the amount of overall saturated fat and calories, which can contribute to obesity and atherosclerosis.

> ***Go fish . . . or chicken!*** Fresh fish is usually abundant in most Mediterranean countries due to their proximity to the sea. Fish is rich in omega-3 fatty acids, which have heart-healthy benefits, such as reducing inflammation, triglycerides, and cholesterol. There are usually plenty of varieties of fish to choose from, including salmon, mackerel, herring, trout, sardines, and albacore tuna—all very high in omega-3 fatty acids. Chicken is also used in place of red meat because it has lower amounts of saturated fat and cholesterol.

> ***Go nuts!*** In Mediterranean countries, unsalted nuts are far more likely to be eaten as a snack than potato chips or crackers. Nuts are often included in savory dishes and desserts, too. Pine nuts are used to make homemade pesto, and walnuts are added to bread dough. Like olive oil, nuts are a good source of monounsaturated fats. Plus, they're packed with fiber and protein, and contain a range of vitamins and minerals to support your overall health.

> ***Red, red wine.*** In Mediterranean countries, small amounts of alcohol are consumed with meals, especially red wine. Much research has been done looking at the specific heart benefits of this alcoholic drink. In particular, red wine contains antioxidants called flavonoids, which may prevent the buildup of fatty deposits within the arteries' walls. The American Heart Association recommends an average of one to two drinks a day (4 ounces per drink) for men and one drink a day for women.

> ***Spice it up.*** Garlic and herbs are used in abundance in Mediterranean dishes and undoubtedly help food taste fabulous. Commonly used herbs and spices in this diet include anise, basil, bay leaf, cumin, fennel, lavender, marjoram, mint, oregano, parsley, pepper, rosemary, sumac, tarragon, and

thyme. Together with fresh herbs, garlic is a great way to add flavor to food without the need to add salt—cutting down on salt can help lower blood pressure, which is a risk factor for heart disease.

> **Do dairy.** In general, full-fat dairy products, such as whole milk and cheese, tend to be eaten in smaller amounts in Mediterranean countries, helping keep intake of saturated fat down. Furthermore, traditional cheeses, such as feta cheese or goat cheese, tend to be lower in fat than traditional hard cheeses, such as Cheddar. Also, yogurt tends to be eaten more frequently and in different dishes, such as tzatziki; as dessert mixed with honey and fruit; or stirred into savory dishes to add a creamy texture. In addition to dairy, eggs are also eaten regularly, but egg yolks should be limited to a maximum of 4 per week to control saturated fat. Egg whites, however, can be eaten in unlimited amounts.

> **Reduced red meat.** Red meat tends to be eaten less frequently in Mediterranean countries, and it is thought to contribute to the lower rates of heart disease. A National Cancer Institute study of 500,000 people found that those who ate the red meat daily, or the most, were 30 percent more likely to die of any cause during a 10-year period than were those who ate less red meat. Sausage, luncheon meat, and other processed meats also increased the risk. If feasible, choose lean red meat and limit each serving to a 3-ounce portion of beef, pork, lamb, and veal, three to four times per month.

> **Peas in a pod.** The Mediterranean diet emphasizes the importance of legumes—any plant that develops seeds lined in a pod that includes more than one seed. Beans, lentils, peas, and snap peas fall into this category. Legumes are also very rich in protein and fiber.

The Mediterranean Diet Pyramid

Scientific research has shown adopting the Mediterranean diet plan, outlined in the pyramid chart below, will provide a host of health benefits, including a lower risk for cancer and improved heart health.

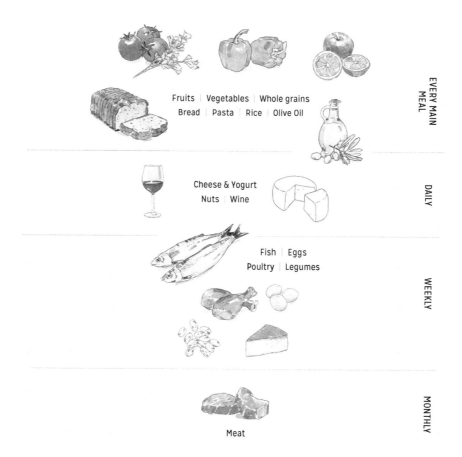

Fruits | Vegetables | Whole grains
Bread | Pasta | Rice | Olive Oil

EVERY MAIN MEAL

Cheese & Yogurt
Nuts | Wine

DAILY

Fish | Eggs
Poultry | Legumes

WEEKLY

Meat

MONTHLY

Mediterranean Lifestyle

Living a Mediterranean lifestyle means more than just eating more fish or adding olive oil to your foods. To get the full experience, you need to embrace the lifestyle—and that means incorporating exercise and relaxation into your daily routine. When I visit my family in Lebanon, I usually get up early and go for a walk around town. An early-morning run or a brisk walk is common practice. Getting enough physical activity is a very important part of the Mediterranean lifestyle. Start with 30 to 60 minutes of moderate exercise 5 times a week. Moderate exercise includes activities such as walking, biking, or swimming.

Another important aspect of this lifestyle is the relaxed pace of family meals. Meals are not rushed in front of the television or computer and shoved down as quickly as possible to get to the next activity. Mealtime is a way to relax with family and friends while enjoying the flavors and aromas of the delicious dishes prepared for you. In some countries, lunch can be a two-hour

Daily Rituals

Not everyone has the luxury to relax for a few hours in the middle of a hectic day, but there are ways to introduce the benefits of the Mediterranean lifestyle into your everyday routine and reduce your daily stress:

> Enjoy lunch outdoors, or at a nearby park with a colleague or friend and truly get to know each other.
> Use some of your lunch hour to enjoy a brisk walk or jog with a friend.
> Turn off your phone or step away from electronics (TV, computer, iPad) during meals.
> Take a walk with your children or friends after dinner.

event. Stores may even close for the break, giving people time to enjoy their lunch, and even squeeze in a nap before returning for their afternoon shift.

Eating any meal is an event, and it's one best shared with family and friends. You talk, laugh, and take your time. Allowing more time to finish your meal gives your brain the ability to register when you're full, and slowing down your eating means you eat less—or rather, just the right amount. It's about enjoying the simple things in life.

CHAPTER 2

Ensuring Your Success

The Mediterranean diet can make a positive change in your life. Remember, it's more of a lifestyle than a diet. It's learning how to enjoy the smaller things in life, and savoring the moments with family and friends at the dinner table. These small steps can take you farther than you might imagine. Leading a healthier lifestyle and living in the moment can make your life more fulfilling and less stressful—not to mention healthier!

Plan Your Week

Everyone loves fresh ingredients, but not everyone has the time to shop for them. A little planning can help. The meal plans, and their recipes, included in this book, are designed not only to give you a taste of the Mediterranean, but also to make this diet easy to follow. There are 4 weeks of meal plans for each version of the Mediterranean diet. I recommend grocery shopping on the weekend so you have everything you need to prepare recipes ahead and have what you need during the week.

Don't forget the Mediterranean diet emphasizes a certain lifestyle, which plays an important supporting role to the diet. Physical activity, fresh air, and relaxed, leisurely meals enjoyed with family and friends are part of the Mediterranean prescription. Plan your meals—and your week with family and friends—in advance. Remember, the Mediterranean diet is about moderation, not elimination, which makes sticking to it easier than other diets.

Manage Your Portions

While the Mediterranean diet is rich in colorful and healthy foods, it also encourages portion control. I have noticed that my patients tend to focus so much on counting calories, they stop caring about the quality of calories and only look at the quantity. While calories are important, the type of calories matters more. Consuming foods with little or no nutritional value can actually lead to overeating. The Mediterranean diet offers nutrient-dense foods that contain a lot of vitamins, minerals, and fiber that have a lot of nutritional value, all while helping you stay full. If you follow basic portion control, counting calories becomes unnecessary. Following are some guidelines to help you stay on track.

A Hand in Portion Control

It can be difficult to tell if the portions we are eating are the right serving size to meet our nutritional needs. To keep from over- or undereating, use these easy-to-follow guidelines as a general estimate.

HAND SYMBOL	EQUIVALENT	FOODS	CALORIES
	Fist 1 cup	Rice, pasta Fruit Veggies	200 75 40
	Palm 3 oz	Meat Fish Poultry	160 160 160
	Handful 1 oz	Nuts Raisins	170 85
	Thumb 1 oz	Peanut Butter Hard Cheese	170 100

Kitchen Staples

We are all more likely to cook and eat at home often with a well-stocked pantry to turn to, and keeping it stocked with staple Mediterranean ingredients helps you adhere to the Mediterranean diet and lifestyle more easily. Remember, it takes time to adjust to anything new, so make it easy on yourself. Take regular inventory at first, and refill items you use most frequently. With time, the Mediterranean diet will become like second nature and you won't even have to keep that list. To get you started in the meantime, here is a basic master grocery list of staples used in all four variations of the Mediterranean diet plans.

10 Key Ingredients

Almonds

Almonds have been heavily researched for their health benefits, specifically for their ability to lower cholesterol and promote weight loss relative to lower-fat diets. Although almonds are typically consumed in their raw form, they are extremely versatile and frequently used in Mediterranean cooking.

Chickpeas

Chickpeas offer benefits like healthy filling doses of fiber. Studies have found that fiber can help manage diabetes, prevent colon cancer, and reduce heart disease risk. Eaten daily, combined with grains and starches, chickpeas provide high-protein value along with folate, calcium, iron, and zinc.

Couscous

A whole grain, couscous retains its fiber, magnesium, vitamin E, and other antioxidant phytochemicals. It is digested more slowly and produces gentler rises in glucose and insulin. Diets rich in whole grains may protect against heart disease, diabetes, and other chronic diseases. Enjoy couscous as a side to fish or beans. You can also add it to your salad to boost the nutrition.

Eggplant

Eggplant contains fiber and potassium. Eggplant has chlorogenic acid, a compound concentrated in eggplant skin, which may have antiviral and cancer-fighting properties. Eggplant can be cooked using several methods, such as frying, stir-frying, grilling, broiling, baking, and roasting.

Garlic

Garlic is great for building up the immune system. It contains high levels of antioxidants, including vitamin C. Commonly used in Mediterranean cuisine, it's a versatile seasoning that complements most any savory dish. It can be used in sauces, stews, soups, salad dressings, casseroles, breads, and grain dishes.

Lentils

Lentils are packed with fiber, B vitamins, protein, and phytochemicals. They're also economical and can create amazing flavor and texture in your meals. Lentils require no soaking before cooking. Just sort through them, discarding any that are discolored or dirty. Give them a good rinse in a colander, and cook them according to package or recipe directions.

Olive Oil

This oil consists of a high amount of monounsaturated fatty acids, which are considered a healthy dietary fat, as opposed to saturated fats and trans fats. Choose extra-virgin olive oil, the highest-quality olive oil extracted through a process called cold pressing. This process removes the oil using pressure only, so it is not heated. This keeps all of the good-for-you antioxidants and monounsaturated fats in the oil. At the end of cooking, for a burst of flavor, drizzle some extra olive oil over pasta or vegetables.

Sustaining the Mediterranean Diet and Lifestyle: 10 Helpful Tips

Use these helpful tips to help you stay on track while following the Mediterranean diet and lifestyle.

1. *Don't skip breakfast.* Keep yogurt and fruit stocked in your refrigerator to eat on the go.

2. *When dining out, divide your meal in half.* Do this the moment the plate hits the table and pack it up as leftovers.

3. *Keep a supply of chopped vegetables.* Celery, bell peppers, carrots, and cucumbers are perfect for dipping in hummus.

4. *Visit your local farmers' market.* This will keep your refrigerator stocked with locally grown, seasonal vegetables.

5. *Snack on a handful of nuts or seeds.* Almonds, walnuts, or sunflower seeds are better choices in place of chips, cookies, or other processed foods.

6. *Enjoy fruit for dessert.* You can even add a little sweetness with a drizzle of honey or sprinkle of brown sugar on top. Keep fresh fruit around the house and at work so you have a healthy snack on hand when your stomach begins to growl.

7. *Savor your bites.* Avoid eating in front of the television or while you're answering email. Cherish your time with family and friends at the dinner table.

8. *Get your family involved.* Ask children to help with food preparation. It allows you to spend quality time with one another.

9. *Avoid processed and refined foods.* Minimize, or better yet, eliminate your consumption of packaged foods and sweets.

10. *Switch to whole grains.* Minimally processed grains, such as barley, bulgur, couscous, faro, millet, oats rice, and, polenta, are a central part of the Mediterranean diet.

Rice

Rice contains carbohydrates that give our bodies the energy we need. It provides fast and instant energy, regulates and improves bowel movements, and stabilizes blood sugars. Enjoy a portion of rice as a side dish. Rice can be prepared in various ways using spices, meats, fish, lentils, beans, and vegetables.

Tomatoes

Packed with vitamin C and lycopene, a heart-protective antioxidant that may also help prevent some cancers. Tomatoes are versatile enough to enjoy every day. They're a staple in every cook's larder—fresh, canned, and in paste form.

Common Food Swaps

Here are 10 easy food swaps to help you adapt to a Mediterranean diet and lifestyle.

1. Use olive oil in place of butter.
2. Use herbs and spices in place of salt.
3. Replace mayonnaise with avocado.
4. Replace beer with a glass or two of red wine.
5. Use salmon in place of beef.
6. Instead of snacking on potato chips, choose mixed nuts.
7. Use fresh fruit instead of jam or jelly.
8. Swap rice or bread for legumes.
9. Replace white rice with bulgur wheat or quinoa.
10. Snack on hummus with vegetables instead of cakes or cookies.

Yogurt

Great for cultivating friendly intestinal bacteria, yogurt is also rich in calcium, vitamin B_2, vitamin B_{12}, potassium, and magnesium. Yogurt is used for salad dressings, such as tzatziki. Choose low-fat yogurt for a quick breakfast or snack, too.

Kitchen Equipment

Mediterranean style cooking doesn't require any fancy or expensive cooking equipment. Here's a basic range of equipment you'll use regularly to perform all kinds of kitchen tasks.

- **Baking dish:** Having a couple sizes of an all-purpose version that can go straight from oven to table to refrigerator or freezer saves the extra work of transferring and storing the contents.

- **Chef's knife:** A chef's knife is an all-purpose tool used for chopping, cutting, slicing, and dicing.

- **Chopping board:** The partner to the chef's knife, a large chopping board is essential in a Mediterranean kitchen.

- **Citrus zester:** The zest and juice of citrus fruits, particularly lemons and limes, really add a delicate zing to dishes, such as pastas, curries, marinades, and salad dressings. This handy tool will save you time and produce the best results.

- **Colander:** Perfect for draining and rinsing vegetables, pasta, and noodles.

- **Food processor:** A food processor is a quick and easy alternative to a traditional mortar and pestle for making pesto, hummus, and curry pastes.

- **Garlic press:** A handy item that makes mincing garlic a breeze.

- **Grater:** Get one with a few grating options for fine, medium, and coarse grating to suit different ingredients, such as cheese, carrots, apples, and cucumbers.

- **Measuring cups:** It's useful to have a glass measuring cup marked with ¼-cup, ½-cup, ¾-cup, and 1-cup amounts (or larger for liquid ingredients), as well as individual measuring cups in these same amounts for dry ingredients.
- **Mixing bowls:** It's useful to have one large bowl, a medium-size bowl, and a small bowl. They can even be used as serving dishes.
- **Mortar and pestle:** Used for grinding and crushing garlic, herbs, nuts, and spices.
- **Pastry brush:** Ideal for brushing olive oil onto bread. It's also useful for brushing chicken or fish with oil before cooking and to baste foods with marinades during grilling.
- **Pepper grinder:** Using a pepper grinder to transform whole peppercorns into freshly ground pepper is more flavorful than pre-ground pepper.
- **Pots and pans:** Heavy-bottomed saucepans are a good choice because the contents can simmer gently on the stove top without burning. A large pot is perfect for making soups, stews, and curries, and doubles as a pasta-cooking pot. A medium-size pot is useful for preparing rice and sauces and boiling eggs, among an endless list of other uses.
- **Sauté pan or skillet:** A large, heavy-bottomed skillet has almost unlimited uses, including sautéing, poaching, and searing foods, such as fish or chicken. Opt for stainless steel or cast iron pans. Avoid nonstick pans coated with Teflon as it can emit toxic fumes.
- **Set of measuring spoons:** A five-piece set will give you a good range for measuring ingredients.

- **Storage containers:** Airtight containers of various sizes serve many purposes. They're great for storing leftovers in the refrigerator or freezer. Use see-through glass or plastic containers to store dried foods, such as cereals, nuts, and spices, so you can see the contents without opening the lid.

- **Vegetable peeler:** A handy utensil for all kinds of peeling tasks. I prefer Y-shaped peelers as they are easier to use.

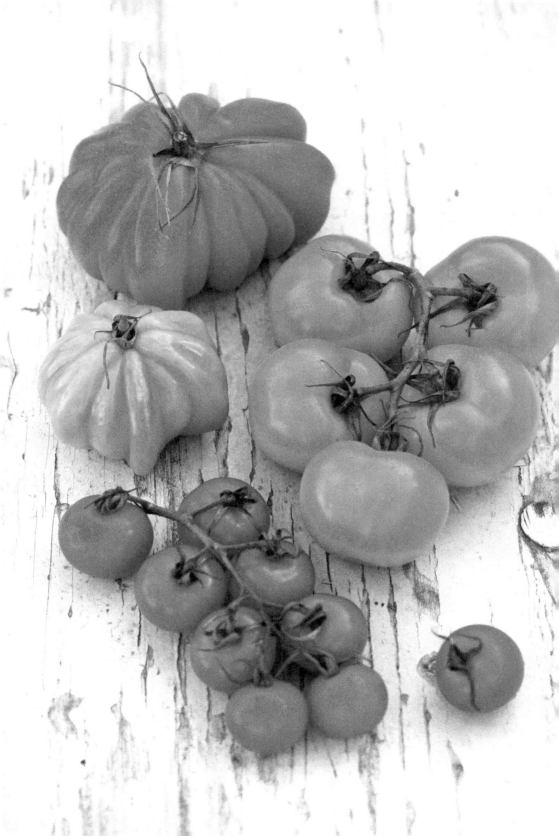

PART TWO

Meal Plans and Recipes

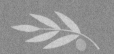

CHAPTER 3

The Right Mediterranean Diet Plan for You

At this point, you probably realize that the Mediterranean diet has many benefits and is good for your health. Choosing which Mediterranean plan is best for you should be fun. The beautiful thing about the Mediterranean diet is that you can switch it up and experience a variety of foods, while still reaping its tremendous health benefits. Those who switch to this style of eating say they'll never eat any other way.

Making the Mediterranean Diet Work for You

There are options for everyone! Whatever your dietary preferences—whether you like meatless, no seafood, traditional items, or are just time-challenged for meal prep, there's a plan for you included here. Just choose which plan fits you best, or try all of them. Each recipe shows which meal plans it works for, taking the guesswork out of meal planning.

All recipes are designed for a family of four, but feel free to make enough for more or reduce the recipe. The meal plans include leftovers, so be sure to look at the whole week ahead and plan accordingly.

- **Traditional Mediterranean Plan:** includes eggs, fish, poultry, beef, a variety of fruits, vegetables, whole grains, beans, soy, tofu, and lentils.

- **Meatless Mediterranean Plan:** your choice if you are a vegetarian or want a meatless meal or side dish. It consists of whole grains, soybeans, tofu, fruits, and vegetables.

- **Seafood-Free Mediterranean Plan:** similar to the Traditional Mediterranean Plan, but it does not include fish. It is still packed with protein and the necessary nutrients for a well-balanced diet.

- **30-Minute Mediterranean Plan:** If you are looking for something quick and easy, this meal plan includes delicious recipes with a Mediterranean flair—all prepared in under 30 minutes.

Becoming Mediterranean

Adopting the Mediterranean lifestyle doesn't require any rigid program or particular cooking skills. Simple, fresh ingredients produce inexpensive and delicious meals. And, regular exercise supports their healthful benefits. Here are a few basic principles to keep in mind when transitioning to a Mediterranean diet.

- Limit the total amount of fat you eat (including heart-healthy fats) to 20 to 35 percent of the total calories you eat. If you eat about 2,000 calories per day, your fat intake can be between 50 and 75 grams (g) per day. Look for foods with heart-healthy fats and essential fatty acids with omega-3 and omega-6, such as seafood and olive oil.
- Get 20 to 30 grams of dietary fiber per day. Fruits, vegetables, whole grains, and dried beans are good sources of fiber.
- Eat more plant-based meals, using beans and soy foods for protein.
- Eat fish or chicken breast twice per week.
- Enjoy dairy products, such as milk, cheese, and yogurt, and try to eat 3 servings per day.
- Opt for whole grains, such as brown rice and those found in whole-grain bread, rather than refined grains.
- Consume more fruits and vegetables. Aim for 5 cups of fruits and vegetables per day.

The Traditional Mediterranean Plan

The common characteristics of the Traditional Mediterranean Plan include heart-healthy ingredients, such as fruits, vegetables, grains, nuts, seeds, and legumes. Monounsaturated fats from olive oil are high in the diet, along with omega-3 fatty acids from fish. Dairy and red meat are consumed in moderation, while chicken and seafood are preferred forms of meat protein. Egg consumption can vary, up to four times a week, contributing a source of fat. Red wine can also be consumed in small amounts.

Over the next four weeks, you'll entice your senses with the blend of fresh ingredients included in traditional Mediterranean recipes. This plan features various combinations of simple ingredients to create mouthwatering dishes that will benefit your health as well as your taste buds. Whether you're looking for an appetizing salad including grains, fresh greens, and an olive oil–based dressing, or a nutrient-dense chicken pilaf with crunchy roasted nuts and traditional spices, grab a glass of red wine and enjoy the fine dining of the Mediterranean.

Monday

Breakfast: Barley Porridge
(double), page 65
Lunch: Cucumber-Yogurt
Salad, page 91
Dinner: Beef Patties (Kefta)
(double), page 225

Tuesday

Breakfast: Leftover Barley
Porridge, page 65
Lunch: Leftover Beef Patties
(Kefta), page 225
Dinner: Chicken Shepherd's
Pie, page 198

Wednesday

Breakfast: Mango-Pear
Smoothie, page 62
Lunch: Leftover Chicken
Shepherd's Pie, page 198
Dinner: Hearty Fish
Chowder, page 182

Thursday

Breakfast: Zucchini Fritters
(Ejjeh), page 67
Lunch: Leftover Hearty Fish
Chowder, page 182
Dinner: Green Bean Stew
(Lubya bi-Zayt), page 160

Friday

Breakfast: Strawberry–Chia
Seed Pudding, page 233
Lunch: Ratatouille (double), page 146
Dinner: Pistachio-Crusted
Sole, page 175

Saturday

Breakfast: Scrambled Eggs with
Ground Beef and Onions, page 76
Lunch: Leftover Ratatouille, page 146
Dinner: Macaroni with Milk
(Macaroni bil-Halib), page 127

Sunday

Breakfast: Pumpkin-Gingerbread
Smoothie, page 64
Lunch: Leftover Macaroni with Milk
(Macaroni bil-Halib) page 127
Dinner: Roasted Turkey Breast
with Herbs and Garlic, page 204

Suggested Snacks

Greek yogurt with fresh
strawberries
Celery, cucumber, and carrot sticks
Multigrain crackers
Chili Kale Chips, page 111
Herbed Yogurt Dip, page 113

Monday

Breakfast: Scrambled Eggs with Ground Beef and Onions, page 76

Lunch: Cucumber-Yogurt Salad, page 91

Dinner: Trout with Wilted Greens, page 174

Tuesday

Breakfast: Mango-Pear Smoothie, page 62

Lunch: Lebanese Bread Salad (Fattoush), page 94

Dinner: Green Bean Stew (Lubya bi-Zayt), page 160

Wednesday

Breakfast: Zucchini Fritters (Ejjeh), page 67

Lunch: Lebanese Bread Salad (Fattoush), page 94

Dinner: Chicken Florentine Casserole, page 188

Thursday

Breakfast: Pumpkin-Gingerbread Smoothie, page 64

Lunch: Leftover Chicken Florentine Casserole, page 188

Dinner: Beef Patties (Kefta) (double), page 225

Friday

Breakfast: Crustless Sun-Dried Tomato Quiche, page 70

Lunch: Leftover Beef Patties (Kefta), page 225

Dinner: Macaroni with Milk (Macaroni bil-Halib), page 127

Saturday

Breakfast: Bircher Muesli, page 66

Lunch: Leftover Macaroni with Milk (Macaroni bil-Halib), page 127

Dinner: Hearty Fish Chowder, page 182

Sunday

Breakfast: Bircher Muesli, page 66

Lunch: Leftover Hearty Fish Chowder, page 182

Dinner: Herb-Rubbed Pork Tenderloin, page 214

Suggested Snacks

Watermelon slices

Multigrain tortilla with peanut butter

Cherry tomatoes and celery sticks

Seed and Nut Snack Bars, page 114

Hummus, page 112

WEEK

2

TRADITIONAL

Monday

Breakfast: Barley Porridge (double), page 65

Lunch: Leftover Herb-Rubbed Pork Tenderloin, page 214

Dinner: Beef Patties (Kefta), page 225

Tuesday

Breakfast: Leftover Barley Porridge, page 65

Lunch: Leftover Beef Patties (Kefta), page 225

Dinner: Green Bean Stew (Lubya bi-Zayt), page 160

Wednesday

Breakfast: Zucchini Fritters (Ejjeh), page 67

Lunch: Edamame-Avocado Salad, page 88

Dinner: Pistachio-Crusted Sole, page 175

Thursday

Breakfast: Citrus Polenta, page 240

Lunch: Cucumber–Yogurt Salad, page 91

Dinner: Chicken Shepherd's Pie, page 198

Friday

Breakfast: Mango–Pear Smoothie, page 62

Lunch: Leftover Chicken Shepherd's Pie, page 198

Dinner: Macaroni with Milk (Macaroni bil-Halib), page 127

Saturday

Breakfast: Scrambled Eggs with Ground Beef and Onions, page 76

Lunch: Leftover Macaroni with Milk (Macaroni bil-Halib), page 127

Dinner: Ratatouille (double), page 146

Sunday

Breakfast: Pumpkin–Gingerbread Smoothie, page 64

Lunch: Leftover Ratatouille, page 146

Dinner: Hearty Fish Chowder, page 182

Suggested Snacks

Greek yogurt with grapes

Celery with almond butter

Almonds

Chili Kale Chips, page 111

Herbed Yogurt Dip, page 113

Monday

Breakfast: Mango-Pear Smoothie, page 62

Lunch: Leftover Hearty Fish Chowder, page 182

Dinner: Chicken Florentine Casserole, page 188

Tuesday

Breakfast: Zucchini Fritters (Ejjeh), page 67

Lunch: Leftover Chicken Florentine Casserole, page 188

Dinner: Beef Patties (Kefta) (double), page 225

Wednesday

Breakfast: Bircher Muesli, page 66

Lunch: Leftover Beef Patties (Kefta), page 225

Dinner: Macaroni with Milk (Macaroni bil-Halib), page 127

Thursday

Breakfast: Pumpkin-Gingerbread Smoothie, page 64

Lunch: Leftover Macaroni with Milk (Macaroni bil-Halib), page 127

Dinner: Trout with Wilted Greens, page 174

Friday

Breakfast: Scrambled Eggs with Ground Beef and Onions, page 76

Lunch: Cucumber-Yogurt Salad, page 91

Dinner: Herb-Rubbed Pork Tenderloin, page 214

Saturday

Breakfast: Barley Porridge (double), page 65

Lunch: Leftover Herb-Rubbed Pork Tenderloin, page 214

Dinner: Turkey Vegetable Chowder, page 86

Sunday

Breakfast: Leftover Barley Porridge, page 65

Lunch: Leftover Turkey Vegetable Chowder, page 86

Dinner: Green Bean Stew (Lubya bi-Zayt), page 160

Suggested Snacks

Mango-Pear Smoothie, page 62

Cashews and raisins

Low-fat ricotta cheese with peaches

Hummus, page 112

Seed and Nut Snack Bars, page 114

WEEK

4

TRADITIONAL

Meatless Mediterranean Plan

The beauty of the Mediterranean diet is its adaptability to various dietary needs. In this Meatless Plan, vegetarians can find comfort in the assortment of recipe options that satisfy their cravings and provide essential nutrients. If you don't consume chicken, beef, or fish—no problem! There are several sources of protein in the Mediterranean diet, including fresh cheeses, hearty nuts and legumes, as well as grains. Naturally, this plan is packed with a variety of produce.

The Meatless Mediterranean Plan includes well-seasoned dishes prepared with herbs, spices, and lots of flavor. Get ready to cook with all kinds of spices, such as cumin, sage, basil, thyme, and paprika—to name a few. Vegetables and fruits, whole grains, legumes, pasta, and olive oil represent the foundation of every meal. Nuts, which provide protein and fiber, are also a great source of heart-healthy fats. Limit your consumption of nuts to about one handful per day. Keep your protein sources focused on dried beans, tofu or tempeh, and some dairy products.

Monday

Breakfast: Artichoke
Frittata, page 72
Lunch: Lebanese Bread Salad
(Fattoush), page 94
Dinner: Classic Colcannon, page 158

Tuesday

Breakfast: Mango-Pear
Smoothie, page 62
Lunch: Lebanese Bread Salad
(Fattoush), page 94
Dinner: White Bean Soup with
Swiss Chard (double), page 84

Wednesday

Breakfast: Zucchini Fritters
(Ejjeh), page 67
Lunch: Leftover White Bean Soup
with Swiss Chard, page 84
Dinner: Macaroni with Milk
(Macaroni bil-Halib), page 127

Thursday

Breakfast: Barley Porridge
(double), page 65
Lunch: Leftover Macaroni with Milk
(Macaroni bil-Halib), page 127
Dinner: Lentil Sesame Patties
(double), page 140

Friday

Breakfast: Leftover Barley
Porridge, page 65
Lunch: Leftover Lentil Sesame
Patties, page 140
Dinner: Ratatouille (double), page 146

Saturday

Breakfast: Ricotta Breakfast
Casserole, page 74
Lunch: Leftover Ratatouille, page 146
Dinner: Green Bean Stew
(Lubya bi-Zayt), page 160

Sunday

Breakfast: Spiced Almond
Pancakes, page 68
Lunch: Cucumber-Yogurt
Salad, page 91
Dinner: Roasted Vegetarian
Lasagna, page 134

Suggested Snacks

Celery, cucumber, and carrot sticks
Watermelon wedges
Plain Greek yogurt with
fresh blueberries
Hummus, page 112
Seed and Nut Snack Bars, page 114

WEEK

1

MEATLESS

MEATLESS

Monday

Breakfast: Mango-Pear
Smoothie, page 62

Lunch: Leftover Roasted
Vegetarian Lasagna, page 134

Dinner: Macaroni with Milk
(Macaroni bil-Halib), page 127

Tuesday

Breakfast: Crustless Sun-Dried
Tomato Quiche, page 70

Lunch: Leftover Macaroni with Milk
(Macaroni bil-Halib), page 127

Dinner: Green Bean Stew
(Lubya bi-Zayt), page 160

Wednesday

Breakfast: Bircher Muesli, page 66

Lunch: Leftover Green Bean Stew
(Lubya bi-Zayt), page 160

Dinner: Lentil Sesame Patties
(double), page 140

Thursday

Breakfast: Zucchini Fritters
(Ejjeh), page 67

Lunch: Leftover Lentil Sesame
Patties, page 140

Dinner: Ratatouille (double), page 146

Friday

Breakfast: Pumpkin-Gingerbread
Smoothie, page 64

Lunch: Lebanese Bread Salad
(Fattoush), page 94

Dinner: Leftover Ratatouille, page 146

Saturday

Breakfast: Spiced Almond
Pancakes, page 68

Lunch: Lebanese Bread Salad
(Fattoush), page 94

Dinner: Classic Colcannon
(double), page 158

Sunday

Breakfast: Artichoke
Frittata, page 72

Lunch: Cucumber-Yogurt
Salad, page 91

Dinner: Leftover Classic
Colcannon, page 158

Suggested Snacks

Cantaloupe wedges

Raisins and almonds

Cherry tomatoes

Seed and Nut Snack Bars, page 114

Herbed Yogurt Dip, page 113

Monday

Breakfast: Barley Porridge, page 65

Lunch: Edamame-Avocado Salad, page 88

Dinner: Green Bean Stew (Lubya bi-Zayt), page 160

Tuesday

Breakfast: Strawberry-Rhubarb Smoothie, page 63

Lunch: Leftover Green Bean Stew (Lubya bi-Zayt), page 160

Dinner: Lentil Sesame Patties (double), page 140

Wednesday

Breakfast: Zucchini Fritters (Ejjeh), page 67

Lunch: Leftover Lentil Sesame Patties, page 140

Dinner: Southwest Pizza, page 118

Thursday

Breakfast: Crustless Sun-Dried Tomato Quiche, page 70

Lunch: Cucumber-Yogurt Salad, page 91

Dinner: Macaroni with Milk (Macaroni bil-Halib), page 127

Friday

Breakfast: Bircher Muesli (double), page 66

Lunch: Leftover Macaroni with Milk (Macaroni bil-Halib), page 127

Dinner: Ratatouille (double), page 146

Saturday

Breakfast: Leftover Bircher Muesli, page 66

Lunch: Leftover Ratatouille, page 146

Dinner: Sweet Potato Curry (double), page 142

Sunday

Breakfast: Spiced Almond Pancakes, page 68

Lunch: Leftover Sweet Potato Curry, page 142

Dinner: Classic Colcannon (double), page 158

Suggested Snacks

Low-fat ricotta cheese with grapes

Olives

Cauliflower and broccoli

Chili Kale Chips, page 111

Hummus, page 112

WEEK

3

MEATLESS

4

Monday

Breakfast: Strawberry-Rhubarb
Smoothie, page 63

Lunch: Leftover Classic
Colcannon, page 158

Dinner: Macaroni with Milk
(Macaroni bil-Halib), page 127

Tuesday

Breakfast: Zucchini Fritters
(Ejjeh), page 67

Lunch: Leftover Macaroni with Milk
(Macaroni bil-Halib), page 127

Dinner: Lentil Sesame Patties
(double), page 140

Wednesday

Breakfast: Pumpkin-Gingerbread
Smoothie, page 64

Lunch: Leftover Lentil Sesame
Patties, page 140

Dinner: Green Bean Stew
(Lubya bi-Zayt), page 160

Thursday

Breakfast: Artichoke Frittata
(double), page 72

Lunch: Leftover Green Bean Stew
(Lubya bi-Zayt), page 160

Dinner: Ratatouille (double), page 146

Friday

Breakfast: Leftover Artichoke
Frittata, page 72

Lunch: Lebanese Bread Salad
(Fattoush), page 94

Dinner: Leftover Ratatouille, page 146

Saturday

Breakfast: Spiced Almond
Pancakes, page 68

Lunch: Lebanese Bread Salad
(Fattoush), page 94

Dinner: Caramelized Onion and
Fennel Pizza, page 120

Sunday

Breakfast: Barley Porridge, page 65

Lunch: Cucumber-Yogurt
Salad, page 91

Dinner: Linguine with Cherry
Tomatoes, page 128

Suggested Snacks

Crudité

Apple

Plain Greek yogurt with
fresh strawberries

Chili Kale Chips, page 111

Herbed Yogurt Dip, page 113

Seafood-Free Mediterranean Plan

If you're not keen on fish or perhaps you have an allergy to it, this is the Mediterranean diet plan for you. With a mixture of grains, garden-fresh vegetables, and legumes, this plan consists of good fat, protein, fiber, vitamins, and minerals that enrich your diet and can benefit any individual looking to decrease his or her intake of processed foods. A good approach to this plan is to include one or two vegetarian meals each week. Other meals can be prepared with lean meat or poultry. The Seafood-Free diet does not lack the essential fatty acids found in seafood, however, because it includes green leafy vegetables, soybeans and soybean oil, hazelnuts, pecans, eggs, and tofu—to name a few sources of this dietary essential.

Beans are a big component of the Seafood-Free Mediterranean Plan and an important source of protein. Many dishes will be drizzled with extra-virgin olive oil, which is very rich in mono-unsaturated fats (healthy fats). You will also gain the benefits of all the wonderful antioxidants rooted in the Traditional Mediterranean Plan, just minus the fish.

Monday

Breakfast: Barley Porridge, page 65

Lunch: Cucumber-Yogurt Salad, page 91

Dinner: Beef Stifado, page 225

Tuesday

Breakfast: Strawberry-Rhubarb Smoothie, page 63

Lunch: Roasted Eggplant Soup, page 82

Dinner: Chopped Kale Tabbouleh (double), page 148

Wednesday

Breakfast: Scrambled Eggs with Ground Beef and Onions, page 76

Lunch: Leftover Chopped Kale Tabbouleh, page 148

Dinner: Herb-Rubbed Pork Tenderloin, page 214

Thursday

Breakfast: Mango-Pear Smoothie, page 62

Lunch: Leftover Herb-Rubbed Pork Tenderloin, page 214

Dinner: Lentil Sesame Patties, page 140

Friday

Breakfast: Bircher Muesli, page 66

Lunch: White Bean Soup with Swiss Chard, page 84

Dinner: Chicken Piccata, page 194

Saturday

Breakfast: Bircher Muesli, page 66

Lunch: Bell Pepper Frittata with Whole-Wheat Penne, page 144

Dinner: Green Bean Stew (Lubya bi-Zayt), page 160

Sunday

Breakfast: Zucchini Fritters (Ejjeh), page 67

Lunch: Leftover Green Bean Stew (Lubya bi-Zayt), page 160

Dinner: Roasted Turkey Breast with Herbs and Garlic (double), page 204

Suggested Snacks

Green grapes

Celery, cucumber, and carrot sticks

Plain Greek yogurt with fresh raspberries

Chili Kale Chips, page 111

Hummus, page 112

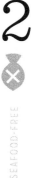
Monday

Breakfast: Strawberry-Rhubarb Smoothie, page 63

Lunch: Leftover Roasted Turkey Breast with Herbs and Garlic, page 204

Dinner: Basil–Goat Cheese Sandwich, page 96

Tuesday

Breakfast: Zucchini Fritters (Ejjeh), page 67

Lunch: Cucumber-Yogurt Salad, page 91

Dinner: Beef Patties (Kefta) (double), page 225

Wednesday

Breakfast: Barley Porridge, page 65

Lunch: Leftover Beef Patties (Kefta), page 225

Dinner: Green Bean Stew (Lubya bi-Zayt), page 160

Thursday

Breakfast: Mango-Pear Smoothie, page 62

Lunch: Green Bean Stew (Lubya bi-Zayt), page 160

Dinner: Herb-Rubbed Pork Tenderloin, page 214

Friday

Breakfast: Bircher Muesli, page 66

Lunch: Leftover Herb-Rubbed Pork Tenderloin, page 214

Dinner: Chopped Kale Tabbouleh (double), page 148

Saturday

Breakfast: Scrambled Eggs with Ground Beef and Onions, page 76

Lunch: Leftover Chopped Kale Tabbouleh, page 148

Dinner: Macaroni with Milk (Macaroni bil-Halib), page 127

Sunday

Breakfast: Spiced Almond Pancakes, page 68

Lunch: Leftover Macaroni with Milk (Macaroni bil-Halib), page 127

Dinner: Lentil Sesame Patties (double), page 140

Suggested Snacks

Almonds and raisins

Watermelon slices

Cauliflower and broccoli

Herbed Yogurt Dip, page 113

Seed and Nut Snack Bars, page 114

Monday

Breakfast: Strawberry-Rhubarb
Smoothie, page 63

Lunch: Leftover Lentil Sesame
Patties, page 140

Dinner: Herb-Rubbed Pork
Tenderloin, page 214

Tuesday

Breakfast: Bircher Muesli, page 66

Lunch: Roasted Eggplant
Soup, page 82

Dinner: Leftover Herb-Rubbed
Pork Tenderloin, page 214

Wednesday

Breakfast: Mango-Pear
Smoothie, page 62

Lunch: White Bean Soup with
Swiss Chard, page 84

Dinner: Chicken Piccata, page 194

Thursday

Breakfast: Scrambled Eggs with
Ground Beef and Onions, page 76

Lunch: Leftover White Bean Soup
with Swiss Chard, page 84

Dinner: Chopped Kale Tabbouleh
(double), page 148

Friday

Breakfast: Barley Porridge, page 65

Lunch: Leftover Chopped Kale
Tabbouleh, page 148

Dinner: Beef Stifado, page 226

Saturday

Breakfast: Spiced Almond
Pancakes, page 68

Lunch: Cucumber-Yogurt
Salad, page 91

Dinner: Green Bean Stew
(Lubya bi-Zayt), page 160

Sunday

Breakfast: Zucchini Fritters
(Ejjeh), page 67

Lunch: Leftover Green Bean Stew
(Lubya bi-Zayt), page 160

Dinner: Savory Turkey Meatballs
(double), page 203

Suggested Snacks

Celery with peanut butter

Low-fat ricotta cheese
with red grapes

Cantaloupe

Hummus, page 112

Seed and Nut Snack Bars, page 114

Monday

Breakfast: Bircher Muesli, page 66

Lunch: Leftover Savory Turkey Meatballs, page 203

Dinner: Lentil Sesame Patties, page 140

Tuesday

Breakfast: Bircher Muesli, page 66

Lunch: Cucumber-Yogurt Salad, page 91

Dinner: Beef Patties (Kefta) (double), page 225

Wednesday

Breakfast: Strawberry-Rhubarb Smoothie, page 63

Lunch: Leftover Beef Patties (Kefta), page 225

Dinner: Chopped Kale Tabbouleh (double), page 148

Thursday

Breakfast: Zucchini Fritters (Ejjeh), page 67

Lunch: Leftover Chopped Kale Tabbouleh, page 148

Dinner: Herb-Rubbed Pork Tenderloin, page 214

Friday

Breakfast: Mango-Pear Smoothie, page 62

Lunch: Leftover Herb-Rubbed Pork Tenderloin, page 214

Dinner: Bell Pepper Frittata with Whole-Wheat Penne, page 144

Saturday

Breakfast: Scrambled Eggs with Ground Beef and Onions, page 76

Lunch: Basil–Goat Cheese Sandwich, page 96

Dinner: Green Bean Stew (Lubya bi-Zayt), page 160

Sunday

Breakfast: Spiced Almond Pancakes, page 68

Lunch: Leftover Green Bean Stew (Lubya bi-Zayt), page 160

Dinner: Chicken Piccata, page 194

Suggested Snacks

Apple with almond butter

Cherry tomatoes

Hardboiled egg

Chili Kale Chips, page 111

Pumpkin-Gingerbread Smoothie, page 64

30-Minute Mediterranean Plan

Lack of time is a major reason many of us forgo eating health-fully. More often than not, simply not having enough time to cook healthier foods leads us to reach for fast, easy, and processed foods. Unfortunately, these foods are made with higher amounts of fat, sodium, and sugar. They are also low in vitamins and minerals, meaning that eating too much of them can affect your waistline—and your health.

You can still reap the benefits of the Mediterranean diet without spending hours in the kitchen. The 30-Minute Mediterranean Plan is just that—if you are looking for quick and easy recipes, keep reading. The recipes included in this meal plan consist of the staples from the Traditional Mediterranean diet and only require 30 minutes or less to prepare.

Beans are a big component of this plan, as is the finishing drizzle of olive oil. Simple and nutritious salads are created using a variety of fruits and vegetables, as well as legumes and grains steamed with herbs and spices. Easy cooking methods combined with the nutritious foods in these recipes will leave you satisfied, with extra time on your hands to relax or spend time with family and friends.

Monday

Breakfast: Scrambled Eggs with Ground Beef and Onions, page 76

Lunch: Summer Vegetable Chicken Wraps, page 98

Dinner: Butternut Squash and White Bean Pilaf, page 138

Tuesday

Breakfast: Mango-Pear Smoothie, page 62

Lunch: Leftover Butternut Squash and White Bean Pilaf, page 138

Dinner: Golden Chicken with Cucumber-Yogurt Sauce (double), page 190

Wednesday

Breakfast: Bircher Muesli (double), page 66

Lunch: Leftover Golden Chicken with Cucumber-Yogurt Sauce, page 190

Dinner: Linguine with Tomato Clam Sauce, page 130

Thursday

Breakfast: Leftover Bircher Muesli, page 66

Lunch: Edamame-Avocado Salad, page 88

Dinner: Beef Patties (Kefta) (double), page 225

Friday

Breakfast: Strawberry-Rhubarb Smoothie, page 63

Lunch: Leftover Beef Patties (Kefta), page 225

Dinner: Southwest Pizza, page 118

Saturday

Breakfast: Zucchini Fritters (Ejjeh), page 67

Lunch: Cucumber-Yogurt Salad, page 91

Dinner: Pistachio-Crusted Sole, page 175

Sunday

Breakfast: Spiced Almond Pancakes, page 68

Lunch: Artichoke Frittata, page 72

Dinner: Beef Sirloin Veggie Kebabs (double), page 222

Suggested Snacks

Celery, cucumber, and carrot sticks

Plain Greek yogurt with fresh blueberries

Almonds

Chili Kale Chips, page 111

Herbed Yogurt Dip, page 113

WEEK

1

30-MINUTES

Monday

Breakfast: Scrambled Eggs with Ground Beef and Onions, page 76

Lunch: Leftover Beef Sirloin Veggie Kebabs, page 222

Dinner: Spinach-Feta Chicken Burgers (double), page 202

Tuesday

Breakfast: Strawberry-Rhubarb Smoothie, page 63

Lunch: Leftover Spinach-Feta Chicken Burgers, page 202

Dinner: Trout with Wilted Greens, page 174

Wednesday

Breakfast: Zucchini Fritters (Ejjeh), page 67

Lunch: Summer Vegetable Chicken Wraps, page 98

Dinner: Butternut Squash and White Bean Pilaf, page 138

Thursday

Breakfast: Mango-Pear Smoothie, page 62

Lunch: Leftover Butternut Squash and White Bean Pilaf, page 138

Dinner: Artichoke Frittata, page 72

Friday

Breakfast: Bircher Muesli (double), page 66

Lunch: Edamame-Avocado Salad, page 88

Dinner: Angel Hair with Asparagus-Kale Pesto, page 131

Saturday

Breakfast: Leftover Bircher Muesli, page 66

Lunch: Cucumber-Yogurt Salad, page 91

Dinner: Beef Patties (Kefta) (double), page 225

Sunday

Breakfast: Spiced Almond Pancakes, page 68

Lunch: Leftover Beef Patties (Kefta), page 225

Dinner: Savory Turkey Meatballs (double), page 203

Suggested Snacks

Red and yellow bell pepper strips

Watermelon slices

Cashews

Hummus, page 112

Seed and Nut Snack Bars, page 114

Monday

Breakfast: Citrus Polenta, page 240

Lunch: Leftover Savory Turkey Meatballs, page 203

Dinner: Pistachio-Crusted Sole, page 175

Tuesday

Breakfast: Mango-Pear Smoothie, page 62

Lunch: Edamame-Avocado Salad, page 88

Dinner: Golden Chicken with Cucumber-Yogurt Sauce (double), page 190

Wednesday

Breakfast: Scrambled Eggs with Ground Beef and Onions, page 76

Lunch: Leftover Golden Chicken with Cucumber-Yogurt Sauce, page 190

Dinner: Beef Patties (Kefta) (double), page 225

Thursday

Breakfast: Strawberry-Rhubarb Smoothie, page 63

Lunch: Leftover Beef Patties (Kefta), page 225

Dinner: Lebanese Bread Salad (Fattoush), page 94

Friday

Breakfast: Bircher Muesli, page 66

Lunch: Lebanese Bread Salad (Fattoush), page 94

Dinner: Broiled Portobello Mushroom Burgers with Goat Cheese, page 156

Saturday

Breakfast: Spiced Almond Pancakes, page 68

Lunch: Cucumber-Yogurt Salad, page 91

Dinner: Beef Sirloin Veggie Kebabs (double), page 222

Sunday

Breakfast: Zucchini Fritters (Ejjeh), page 67

Lunch: Leftover Beef Sirloin Veggie Kebabs, page 222

Dinner: Pan-Seared Haddock with Olive-Tomato Sauce (double), page 178

Suggested Snacks

Apple

Low-fat ricotta cheese with grapes

Hardboiled egg

Mango-Pear Smoothie, page 62

Seed and Nut Snack Bars, page 114

WEEK

3

30-MINUTES

Monday

Breakfast: Scrambled Eggs with Ground Beef and Onions, page 76

Lunch: Leftover Pan-Seared Haddock with Olive-Tomato Sauce, page 178

Dinner: Southwest Pizza, page 118

Tuesday

Breakfast: Strawberry-Rhubarb Smoothie, page 63

Lunch: Edamame-Avocado Salad, page 88

Dinner: Spinach-Feta Chicken Burgers (double), page 202

Wednesday

Breakfast: Bircher Muesli (double), page 66

Lunch: Leftover Spinach-Feta Chicken Burgers, page 202

Dinner: Butternut Squash and White Bean Pilaf, page 138

Thursday

Breakfast: Leftover Bircher Muesli, page 66

Lunch: Butternut Squash and White Bean Pilaf, page 138

Dinner: Beef Patties (Kefta) (double), page 225

Friday

Breakfast: Mango-Pear Smoothie, page 62

Lunch: Leftover Beef Patties (Kefta), page 225

Dinner: Angel Hair with Asparagus-Kale Pesto, page 131

Saturday

Breakfast: Zucchini Fritters (Ejjeh), page 67

Lunch: Cucumber-Yogurt Salad, page 91

Dinner: Trout with Wilted Greens, page 174

Sunday

Breakfast: Spiced Almond Pancakes, page 68

Lunch: Artichoke Frittata, page 72

Dinner: Beef Sirloin Veggie Kebabs, page 222

Suggested Snacks

Cottage cheese with fresh raspberries

Carrot sticks

Pistachios

Chili Kale Chips, page 111

Herbed Yogurt Dip, page 113

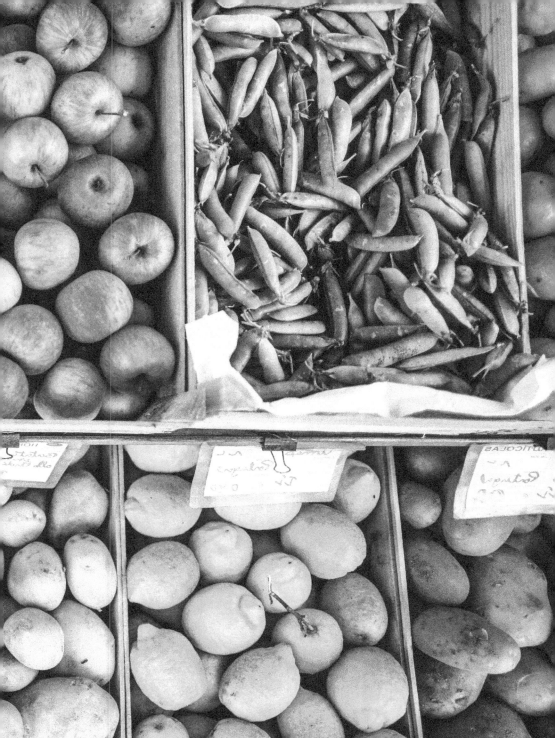

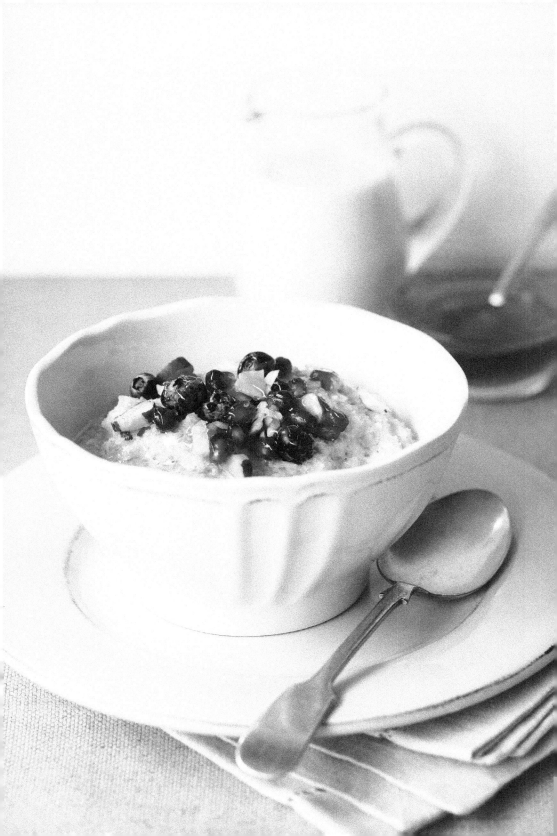

CHAPTER 4

Breakfast

Mango-Pear Smoothie

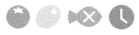

Mango adds a delightful yellow hue and luscious flavor to this silky, almost decadent, smoothie. This bright, fragrant fruit is a wonderful source of vitamins A and C, as well as copper, potassium, and fiber, which means it supports healthy skin and vision while fighting cancer.

1 ripe pear, cored and chopped

½ mango, peeled, pitted, and chopped

1 cup chopped kale

½ cup plain Greek yogurt

2 ice cubes

1. In a blender, purée the pear, mango, kale, and yogurt.
2. Add the ice and blend until thick and smooth. Pour the smoothie into a glass and serve cold.

Substitution tip: Apples can be used instead of pear. For some extra fiber, leave the skin on the fruit. Wash the skin thoroughly, though, to remove any pesticide residue if your apples are not organic.

PER SERVING Calories: 293; Total Fat: 8g; Saturated Fat: 5g; Carbohydrates: 53g; Fiber: 7g; Protein: 8g

Strawberry-Rhubarb Smoothie

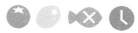

SERVES 1 / PREP TIME: 5 MINUTES / COOK TIME: 3 MINUTES

While perusing the produce at your local grocery store, you might think that the bundles of rhubarb look a little like reddish celery rather than an ingredient used in pies and cakes. Tart rhubarb is cooked, in most cases, like a fruit, but it is actually a vegetable. It is a healthy addition to a breakfast smoothie because rhubarb is very high in vitamin K, lutein, and calcium.

1 rhubarb stalk, chopped

1 cup sliced fresh strawberries

½ cup plain Greek yogurt

2 tablespoons honey

Pinch ground cinnamon

3 ice cubes

1. Place a small saucepan filled with water over high heat and bring to a boil. Add the rhubarb and boil for 3 minutes. Drain and transfer the rhubarb to a blender.

2. Add the strawberries, yogurt, honey, and cinnamon and pulse the mixture until it is smooth.

3. Add the ice and blend until thick, with no ice lumps remaining. Pour the smoothie into a glass and enjoy cold.

Ingredient tip: *Rhubarb leaves contain a compound called oxalic acid, which is toxic—use only the stems of the plant in your recipes.*

PER SERVING Calories: 295; Total Fat: 8g; Saturated Fat: 5g; Carbohydrates: 56g; Fiber: 4g; Protein: 6g

Pumpkin-Gingerbread Smoothie

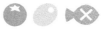

SERVES 1 / PREP TIME: 5 MINUTES, PLUS 1 HOUR OR OVERNIGHT SOAKING

Soak the chia seeds in the refrigerator overnight, and they'll be ready for your smoothie by morning. Chia seeds are incredibly absorbent, sucking up about 10 times their weight in liquid. If you are trying to reach weight-loss goals, stabilize blood sugar, or just support a healthy digestive system, include chia seeds in your diet regularly.

1 cup unsweetened almond milk

2 teaspoons chia seeds

1 banana

½ cup canned pure pumpkin

¼ teaspoon ground cinnamon

¼ teaspoon ground ginger

Pinch ground nutmeg

1. In a small bowl, mix the almond milk and chia seeds. Soak the seeds for at least 1 hour. Transfer the seeds to a blender.

2. Add the banana, pumpkin, cinnamon, ginger, and nutmeg.

3. Blend until smooth. Pour the smoothie into a glass and serve.

Substitution tip: *Cooked sweet potato or butternut squash works as an alternative if you do not have pumpkin handy.*

PER SERVING Calories: 200; Total Fat: 5g; Saturated Fat: 1g; Carbohydrates: 41g; Fiber: 10g; Protein: 5g

Barley Porridge

SERVES 4 / PREP TIME: 5 MINUTES / COOK TIME: 25 MINUTES

Porridge is usually composed of oats, but nutty tasting, slightly chewy barley is a stellar variation. Use hulled barley for this recipe, which can be found in the bulk section of most grocery stores if you want to save a little money. Barley can help fight breast cancer and heart disease, as well as type 2 diabetes, because it is very high in fiber, manganese, selenium, and vitamin B_1.

1 cup barley	½ cup blueberries
1 cup wheat berries	½ cup pomegranate seeds
2 cups unsweetened almond milk, plus more for serving	½ cup hazelnuts, toasted and chopped
2 cups water	¼ cup honey

1. In a medium saucepan over medium-high heat, place the barley, wheat berries, almond milk, and water. Bring to a boil, reduce the heat to low, and simmer for about 25 minutes, stirring frequently until the grains are very tender.

2. Top each serving with almond milk, 2 tablespoons of blueberries, 2 tablespoons of pomegranate seeds, 2 tablespoons of hazelnuts, and 1 tablespoon of honey.

Substitution tip: *Bulgur is a healthy protein and fiber-packed substitution for the barley in this hot breakfast. Bulgur is a cracked, partially cooked wheat kernel.*

PER SERVING Calories: 354; Total Fat: 8g; Saturated Fat: 1g; Carbohydrates: 63g; Fiber: 10g; Protein: 11g

Bircher Muesli

SERVES 4 / PREP TIME: 10 MINUTES, PLUS 6 HOURS OR OVERNIGHT SOAKING

Bircher muesli first made its appearance around 1900 as a breakfast dish at Dr. Bircher's Swiss health clinic, which promoted healthy, holistic eating. Soaking the ingredients is crucial to create a soft texture and combine the various flavors. Try adding a little grated apple, instead of banana, if you want a more traditional muesli.

1½ cups rolled oats

½ cup unsweetened
  shredded coconut

2 cups unsweetened almond milk

2 bananas, mashed

½ cup chopped almonds

½ cup raisins

½ teaspoon ground cinnamon

1. In a large sealable container, stir together the oats, coconut, and almond milk until well combined. Refrigerate the mixture to soak overnight.

2. In the morning, stir in the banana, almonds, raisins, and cinnamon to serve.

Substitution tip: If you do not want a vegetarian breakfast, use 2 percent milk instead of nut milk.

PER SERVING Calories: 397; Total Fat: 18g; Saturated Fat: 8g; Carbohydrates: 55g; Fiber: 10g; Protein: 9g

Zucchini Fritters (Ejjeh)

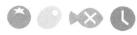

Eggs are very popular in the Middle East, and variations of omelets are prepared often. Zucchini fritters are similar to an omelet and can be fried or baked.

2 zucchini, peeled and grated

1 sweet onion, finely diced

1 cup chopped fresh parsley

2 garlic cloves, minced

½ teaspoon sea salt

½ teaspoon freshly ground black pepper

½ teaspoon ground allspice

4 large eggs

2 tablespoons extra-virgin olive oil

1. Line a plate with paper towels and set aside.

2. In a large bowl, mix the zucchini, onion, parsley, garlic, sea salt, pepper, and allspice.

3. In a medium bowl, beat the eggs and then pour them over the zucchini mixture. Stir to mix.

4. In a large skillet over medium heat, heat the olive oil. Scoop ¼-cup portions of the egg-zucchini mixture into the skillet. Cook until the bottom is set, for about 3 minutes. Flip and cook for 3 minutes more. Transfer the cooked fritters to the paper towel–lined plate. Repeat with the remaining egg-zucchini mixture.

5. Served with pita bread, if desired.

Substitution tip: Don't like zucchini? No problem—use eggplant instead. You can also enjoy these fritters with a side of plain Greek yogurt. They make a delicious combination.

PER SERVING Calories: 103; Total Fat: 8g; Saturated Fat: 2g; Carbohydrates: 5g; Fiber: 1g; Protein: 5g

Spiced Almond Pancakes

SERVES 6 / PREP TIME: 10 MINUTES / COOK TIME: 20 MINUTES

Coconut oil provides a delicate counterpoint taste to the almond flour and is a heart-friendly addition to your breakfast routine. Coconut oil is a saturated fat but is predominantly a medium-chain triglyceride, unlike animal fats, which are long-chain fats. So you can eat coconut oil without worrying about it being stored as fat in your body.

2 cups unsweetened almond milk, at room temperature

½ cup melted coconut oil, plus more for greasing the skillet

2 large eggs, at room temperature

2 teaspoons honey

1½ cups whole-wheat flour

½ cup almond flour

1½ teaspoons baking powder

½ teaspoon baking soda

¼ teaspoon sea salt

¼ teaspoon ground cinnamon

1. In a large bowl, whisk the almond milk, coconut oil, eggs, and honey until blended.

2. In a medium bowl, sift together the whole-wheat flour, almond flour, baking powder, baking soda, sea salt, and cinnamon until well mixed.

3. Add the flour mixture to the milk mixture and whisk until just combined.

4. Grease a large skillet with coconut oil and place it over medium-high heat.

5. Add the pancake batter in ½-cup measures, about 3 for a large skillet. Cook for about 3 minutes until the edges are firm, the bottom is golden, and the bubbles on the surface break. Flip and cook for about 2 minutes more until the other side is golden brown and the pancakes are cooked through. Transfer to a plate and wipe the skillet with a clean paper towel.

6. Regrease the skillet and repeat until the remaining batter is used.

7. Serve the pancakes warm with fresh fruit, if desired.

Cooking tip: *The pancakes can be made ahead. After they cool, keep refrigerated for a cold treat topped with a spoonful of honey. You can also quickly reheat the cooked pancakes in a toaster if you prefer them warm.*

PER SERVING Calories: 286; Total Fat: 17g; Saturated Fat: 12g; Carbohydrates: 27g; Fiber: 1g; Protein: 6g

Crustless Sun-Dried Tomato Quiche

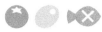

SERVES 4 / PREP TIME: 15 MINUTES / COOK TIME: 25 MINUTES

Quiche is sometimes a ladies-that-lunch dish cradled in a pastry shell that adds calories and fat to the meal. This quiche has no crust, so it is healthier, and the flavor of the ingredients shines through. Sun-dried tomatoes can be found either completely dried or packed in oil. If you use the oil-packed variety, rinse them off completely and pat them dry before adding to the eggs.

6 large eggs

¼ cup goat cheese

2 tablespoons milk

Pinch cayenne pepper

1 teaspoon extra-virgin
  olive oil

2 shallots, finely chopped

½ teaspoon minced garlic

10 sun-dried tomatoes, quartered

1 teaspoon chopped fresh parsley

Pinch sea salt

Pinch freshly ground black pepper

1. Preheat the oven to 375ºF.

2. In a medium bowl, whisk the eggs, goat cheese, milk, and cayenne pepper to blend.

3. Place a 9-inch ovenproof skillet over medium-high heat and add the olive oil.

4. Add the shallots and garlic to the skillet, and sauté for about 2 minutes until tender.

5. Pour in the egg mixture. Scatter the sun-dried tomatoes and parsley evenly over the top.

6. Season the quiche with sea salt and pepper.

7. Cook the quiche, lifting the edges to allow the uncooked egg to flow underneath, for about 3 minutes until the bottom is firm.

8. Place the skillet in the oven and bake for about 20 minutes until the egg is cooked through, golden, and puffy.

Cooking tip: If you have leftover quiche, wrap it in a tortilla the next day for an easy, hearty lunch or breakfast.

PER SERVING Calories: 171; Total Fat: 11g; Saturated Fat: 4g; Carbohydrates: 5g; Fiber: 1g; Protein: 13g

Artichoke Frittata

SERVES 4 / PREP TIME: 5 MINUTES / COOK TIME: 10 MINUTES

Artichokes are sold fresh, and artichoke hearts are sold marinated in oil or packed in water. Use the water-packed variety for this frittata to avoid adding extra oil or changing the texture of the dish. Artichokes are extremely high in fiber, calcium, copper, and many B vitamins, as well as an excellent source of disease-busting antioxidants. Artichokes can help reduce cholesterol, support liver health, and cut your risk of cancer.

8 large eggs

¼ cup grated Asiago cheese

1 tablespoon chopped fresh basil

1 teaspoon chopped
  fresh oregano

Pinch sea salt

Pinch freshly ground black pepper

1 teaspoon extra-virgin
  olive oil

1 teaspoon minced garlic

1 cup canned, water-packed,
  quartered artichoke
  hearts, drained

1 tomato, chopped

1. Preheat the oven to broil.

2. In a medium bowl, whisk the eggs, Asiago cheese, basil, oregano, sea salt, and pepper to blend.

3. Place a large ovenproof skillet over medium-high heat and add the olive oil. Add the garlic and sauté for 1 minute.

4. Remove the skillet from the heat and pour in the egg mixture.

5. Return the skillet to the heat and evenly sprinkle the artichoke hearts and tomato over the eggs.

6. Cook the frittata without stirring for about 8 minutes, or until the center is set.

7. Place the skillet under the broiler for about 1 minute, or until the top is lightly browned and puffed.

8. Cut the frittata into 4 pieces and serve.

Substitution tip: *If you don't need a vegetarian dish, add chopped cooked chicken, cooked shrimp, or smoked salmon to this frittata for extra protein.*

PER SERVING Calories: 199; Total Fat: 13g; Saturated Fat: 5g; Carbohydrates: 5g; Fiber: 2g; Protein: 16g

Ricotta Breakfast Casserole

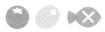

SERVES 4 / PREP TIME: 15 MINUTES / COOK TIME: 25 MINUTES

Casseroles are perfect for times when you want a gorgeous meal without all the fuss and cleanup, such as a family brunch or a holiday morning. Throw together all the ingredients for this dish the night before, and pop the casserole in the oven in the morning right from the refrigerator. Enjoy a leisurely cup of fresh brewed coffee or orange juice instead of slaving over a hot stove or chopping vegetables.

1 teaspoon extra-virgin olive oil

1 zucchini, chopped

1 cup broccoli florets, blanched or steamed

½ cup diced cooked carrots

½ red bell pepper, seeded and diced

8 large eggs

½ cup low-fat ricotta cheese

1 teaspoon chopped fresh basil

1 teaspoon chopped fresh oregano

1 teaspoon chopped fresh chives

Pinch sea salt

Pinch freshly ground black pepper

1. Preheat the oven to 350ºF.

2. Lightly grease an 8-by-8-inch baking dish with olive oil. Evenly distribute the zucchini, broccoli, carrots, and red bell pepper over the bottom of the dish.

3. In a large bowl, whisk together the eggs, ricotta, basil, oregano, chives, sea salt, and pepper. Pour the eggs into the prepared dish over the vegetables.
4. Bake the casserole for about 25 minutes, or until a knife inserted near the center comes out clean.

Substitution tip: Ricotta adds an interesting texture, but you can easily substitute goat cheese, feta cheese, or even plain cottage cheese with equally superb results.

PER SERVING Calories: 220; Total Fat: 14g; Saturated Fat: 5g; Carbohydrates: 7g; Fiber: 2g; Protein: 17g

Scrambled Eggs with Ground Beef and Onions

SERVES 6 / PREP TIME: 5 MINUTES / COOK TIME: 25 MINUTES

This scrambled egg recipe is a delightful way to stretch a little bit of meat, and the sautéed onions add a little pizzazz to the meal. This breakfast item can also be enjoyed with toasted pita bread, if desired. The Mediterranean diet includes a lot of eggs and egg dishes. Frittatas and scrambles are very popular; they are not just for breakfast, either. Egg dishes make great one-dish meals for easy weeknight dinners, too.

½ pound 92% lean ground beef

½ cup diced onion

1 teaspoon ground allspice

1½ teaspoons sea salt

½ teaspoon freshly ground black pepper

6 large eggs

¼ cup milk

1 tablespoon chopped fresh parsley

1. In a large nonstick skillet over medium heat, combine the ground beef and onion. Cook for about 15 minutes until the meat is browned and the onion is softened, stirring occasionally with a wooden spoon to break up the meat.

2. Stir in the allspice, sea salt, and pepper.

3. In a large bowl, whisk the eggs and milk.

4. Reduce the heat to low and pour the egg mixture over the meat. As the eggs begin to set, gently pull the eggs across the pan with an inverted spatula, forming large soft curds. Continue cooking, pulling, lifting, and folding the eggs, until thickened and no visible liquid egg remains. Sprinkle with parsley and serve.

Recipe tip: *For best results, use "lean" beef. To be called "lean," ground beef must be 92% lean, with 8% fat. "Extra lean" ground beef must be 96% lean, with 4% fat.*

PER SERVING Calories: 144; Total Fat: 7g; Saturated Fat: 2g; Carbohydrates: 2g; Fiber: 0g; Protein: 18g

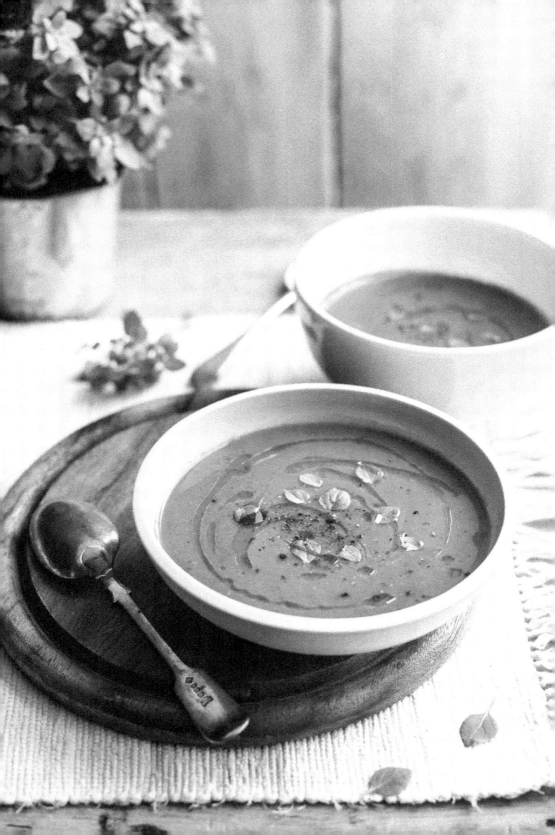

CHAPTER 5

Soups, Salads & Sandwiches

Roasted Bell Pepper and Tomato Soup

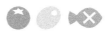

SERVES 4 / PREP TIME: 15 MINUTES / COOK TIME: 30 MINUTES

Tomato soup played a big role in the childhood lunches of many people, although the thin, strangely sweet canned version was probably the one most often eaten. This homemade tomato soup is a totally different culinary experience, featuring a rich, deeply flavored purée with a hint of sweet red pepper. Tomatoes are actually healthier when cooked because an antioxidant found in this food, lycopene, is easier to absorb when tomatoes are heated.

3 tablespoons extra-virgin olive oil, plus extra for finishing (optional)

2 pounds tomatoes, stem ends removed and halved

1 pound red bell peppers, stemmed and seeded

1 sweet onion, peeled and quartered

6 garlic cloves, smashed

2 tablespoons balsamic vinegar

¼ teaspoon sea salt

¼ teaspoon freshly ground black pepper

4 cups vegetable stock or broth

2 tablespoons chopped fresh basil

1. Preheat the oven to 375ºF.

2. Lightly oil a large roasting pan with 1 tablespoon of olive oil.

3. Place the tomatoes and red peppers cut-side down in the roasting pan in a single layer, if possible.

4. Scatter the onion and garlic over the vegetables in the pan.

5. Drizzle the vegetables with the remaining 2 tablespoons of olive oil and the balsamic vinegar, and season them with sea salt and black pepper.

6. Roast the vegetables for about 30 minutes until tender and fragrant. Remove the pan from the oven and let cool for 10 minutes.

7. In a food processor, purée the vegetables in batches with enough stock to thin the soup, as needed.

8. Transfer the puréed batches to a large saucepan over medium heat, and bring the soup to a simmer. Adjust the thickness with more stock, if necessary.

9. Top with the basil and olive oil, if using, and serve.

Ingredient tip: Traditional balsamic vinegar is an Italian culinary treasure. It can be aged for more than 25 years and cost more than $200 per ounce.

PER SERVING Calories: 192; Total Fat: 11g; Saturated Fat: 2g; Carbohydrates: 21g; Fiber: 6g; Protein: 4g

Roasted Eggplant Soup

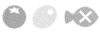

SERVES 4 / PREP TIME: 15 MINUTES, PLUS 30 MINUTES RESTING / COOK TIME: 45 MINUTES

Fans of baba ghanouj *will enjoy the eggplant and tahini combination of flavors in this bowl of steaming soup. Tahini is made from ground sesame seeds and adds an almost luscious, rich, nutty taste. Any type of tahini is packed with vitamins and minerals, but the unhulled product has even more vitamin B and vitamin E, as well as calcium and magnesium.*

2 medium eggplants, halved

1 teaspoon sea salt

1 tablespoon extra-virgin olive oil

1 sweet onion, peeled and diced

1 tablespoon minced garlic

4 cups vegetable stock or broth

2 teaspoons ground cumin

1 teaspoon ground coriander

½ cup heavy (whipping) cream

¼ cup tahini

1 tablespoon chopped fresh cilantro

1. Sprinkle the eggplant halves with sea salt and set aside for 30 minutes.

2. Preheat the oven to 400ºF.

3. Rinse the eggplant halves and place them cut-side down on a baking sheet. Roast the eggplant for about 30 minutes until soft and collapsed. Remove from the oven and scoop out the flesh into a large bowl. Set aside.

4. In a large stockpot over medium-high heat, heat the olive oil.

5. Add the onion and garlic and sauté for about 3 minutes, or until softened.

6. Stir in the vegetable stock, cumin, and coriander, along with the eggplant flesh. Bring to a boil and then reduce the heat to low. Simmer for 10 minutes, stirring frequently.

7. In a food processor or with a handheld immersion blender, purée the soup until smooth, in batches if needed.

8. Stir in the heavy cream and tahini.

9. Garnish the soup with cilantro and serve.

Substitution tip: *Plain Greek yogurt will impart a lovely tangy flavor and add the desired creaminess to this soup if you want to use it instead of heavy (whipping) cream.*

PER SERVING Calories: 294; Total Fat: 17g; Saturated Fat: 5g; Carbohydrates: 33g; Fiber: 17g; Protein: 8g

White Bean Soup with Swiss Chard

SERVES 4 / PREP TIME: 15 MINUTES / COOK TIME: 30 MINUTES

Some soups are just meant to be enjoyed on snowy winter days or crisp autumn nights sitting by a crackling fire. Silky white beans, heaps of vegetables, and a hint of heat from red pepper flakes combine perfectly in a garlicky broth. If you want to freeze a portion, leave out the Swiss chard because it can get mushy. Add it when you reheat the soup.

1 teaspoon extra-virgin olive oil

2 celery stalks, diced

1 sweet onion, peeled and chopped

2 teaspoons minced garlic

6 cups vegetable or chicken stock, or broth

1 (15-ounce) can sodium-free Great Northern beans, drained and rinsed

1 cup diced tomato

2 carrots, peeled and diced

2 cups shredded Swiss chard

1 cup green beans, cut into 1-inch pieces

¼ teaspoon red pepper flakes

Sea salt

Freshly ground black pepper

1. In a medium stockpot over medium-high heat, heat the olive oil.

2. Add the celery, onion, and garlic, and sauté for about 5 minutes until softened.

3. Stir in the stock, beans, tomato, and carrots. Bring to a boil and then reduce the heat to low. Simmer the soup for about 15 minutes until the carrots are tender.

4. Add the Swiss chard, green beans, and red pepper flakes. Simmer for 5 minutes more.

5. Season the soup with sea salt and black pepper before serving.

Ingredient tip: Canned Great Northern beans can be hard to find in grocery stores, but you can soak dried beans and cook the day before you want to make this soup, or substitute another favorite canned variety.

PER SERVING Calories: 168; Total Fat: 3g; Saturated Fat: 0g; Carbohydrates: 29g; Fiber: 10g; Protein: 7g

Turkey Vegetable Chowder

SERVES 6 / PREP TIME: 20 MINUTES / COOK TIME: 45 MINUTES

Holiday meals often feature huge roast turkeys and enough leftover turkey meat for several meals. This soup is an inspired use of both dark and light turkey meat, and you can throw the carcass into a big pot to make authentic turkey stock. Turkey meat can help lower blood sugar levels, and a small 4-ounce portion has more than 30 grams of protein.

1 tablespoon extra-virgin olive oil

1 sweet onion, peeled and chopped

1 tablespoon minced garlic

3 celery stalks, chopped

8 cups chicken or turkey stock, or broth

4 cups chopped cooked turkey meat, dark and white

2 sweet potatoes, peeled and diced

2 carrots, peeled and diced

2 parsnips, peeled and diced

1 teaspoon chopped fresh thyme

¼ teaspoon chopped fresh rosemary

2 cups corn kernels, fresh or frozen

¼ cup water

2 teaspoons cornstarch

Sea salt

Freshly ground black pepper

1. In a large stockpot over medium-high heat, heat the olive oil.

2. Add the onion and garlic and sauté for about 3 minutes until softened.

3. Add the celery and sauté for 2 minutes.

4. Stir in the stock, turkey, sweet potatoes, carrots, parsnips, thyme, and rosemary. Bring to a boil, reduce the heat to low, and simmer for about 30 minutes until the vegetables are tender.

5. Stir in the corn and simmer for 3 minutes.

6. In a small bowl, whisk together the water and cornstarch until smooth.

7. Stir the cornstarch mixture into the hot soup. Cook for about 3 minutes, stirring, until the soup thickens.

8. Season with sea salt and pepper before serving.

Ingredient tip: Organic pasture-raised turkeys are a healthy option because they roam freely and aren't given antibiotics. Never believe a label that states your turkey is grass-fed, because these birds are omnivores.

PER SERVING Calories: 378; Total Fat: 8g; Saturated Fat: 2g; Carbohydrates: 45g; Fiber: 8g; Protein: 32g

Edamame-Avocado Salad

SERVES 4 / PREP TIME: 15 MINUTES, PLUS 1 HOUR CHILLING

If you want to add more protein to your diet, look no further than this pretty, filling salad. Edamame and quinoa are packed with protein, and quinoa is a complete protein because it contains all nine essential amino acids that the body does not produce. Quinoa is often thought to be a grain, but it is actually an ancient seed used for centuries in the Americas.

For the dressing
¼ cup extra-virgin olive oil

2 tablespoons balsamic vinegar

1 teaspoon chopped
  fresh oregano

Sea salt

Freshly ground black pepper

For the salad
1 cup frozen edamame, shelled

1 cup cooked quinoa

1 cup halved cherry tomatoes

½ cup finely chopped red onion

½ English cucumber, diced

½ avocado, diced

2 tablespoons grated
  Parmesan cheese

1 tablespoon chopped
  fresh parsley

To make the dressing

1. In a small bowl, whisk the extra-virgin olive oil, balsamic vinegar, and oregano.

2. Season with sea salt and pepper and set aside.

To make the salad

1. In a large bowl, toss together the edamame, quinoa, tomatoes, onion, cucumber, avocado, and Parmesan cheese until well mixed.

2. Add the dressing and toss to combine.

3. Top with parsley and refrigerate the salad for 1 hour before serving.

Substitution tip: *Edamame are a popular product for vegans looking for good-quality protein. This salad can be made vegan by omitting the Parmesan cheese.*

PER SERVING Calories: 374; Total Fat: 24g; Saturated Fat: 4g; Carbohydrates: 27g; Fiber: 7g; Protein: 14g

Watermelon, Beet, and Radish Salad

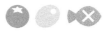

SERVES 4 / PREP TIME: 15 MINUTES PLUS COOLING / COOK TIME: 25 MINUTES

If you could create summer on a plate, it might look very similar to this glorious salad, which features deep greens and lovely shades of red—from the deep maroon of the beets to the pink hue of the watermelon. Watermelon is an excellent source of antioxidants, especially lycopene, which helps reduce blood pressure by improving blood flow.

10 medium beets, peeled and cut into 1-inch chunks

1 teaspoon extra-virgin olive oil

4 cups diced seedless watermelon

5 large radishes, quartered

1 cup shredded kale

1 tablespoon chopped fresh thyme

Juice of 1 lemon

Sea salt

Freshly ground black pepper

1. Preheat the oven to 350°F.

2. In a small bowl, place the beets and olive oil. Toss to coat and transfer the beets to a baking sheet.

3. Roast the beets for about 25 minutes until tender. Transfer to a large bowl and cool them completely.

4. Add the watermelon, radishes, kale, thyme, and lemon juice. Gently toss to combine.

5. Season with sea salt and pepper and serve.

Ingredient tip: Try to purchase watermelon when it is ripe because the antioxidant levels in the fruit start to drop about 2 days after peak ripeness.

PER SERVING Calories: 178; Total Fat: 2g; Saturated Fat: 0g; Carbohydrates: 39g; Fiber: 6g; Protein: 6g

Cucumber-Yogurt Salad

SERVES 4 / PREP TIME: 10 MINUTES

Mint is frequently used in Mediterranean cooking, and blends especially well with fruit and meats. It is also a common ingredient in yogurt sauces. Serve this salad with a meat dish for a superb flavor combination.

5 or 6 small cucumbers, peeled and diced

1 (8-ounce) container plain Greek yogurt

2 garlic cloves, minced

1 tablespoon minced fresh mint

1 teaspoon dried oregano

Sea salt

Freshly ground black pepper

1. In a large bowl, mix the cucumbers, yogurt, garlic, mint, and oregano.

2. Season with sea salt and pepper.

3. Refrigerate the salad for 1 hour before serving for a more refreshing taste.

Ingredient tip: Taste the cucumbers before you make this salad. You don't want them to be bitter.

PER SERVING Calories: 68; Total Fat: 1g; Saturated Fat: 1g; Carbohydrates: 11g; Fiber: 1g; Protein: 4g

Peach and Mixed Green Salad with Chicken

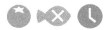

SERVES 4 / PREP TIME: 20 MINUTES

Golden peaches and cooked chicken are accented perfectly by the almost purplish color of fresh blueberries. Blueberries are low in calories and very high in phytonutrients, calcium, potassium, folic acid, vitamin B_1, and antioxidants. Including this superfood regularly in your meals can help lower blood pressure, fight against degenerative diseases, and boost your metabolism.

For the dressing

¼ cup plain Greek yogurt

2 tablespoons honey

2 tablespoons white balsamic vinegar

1 tablespoon extra-virgin olive oil

2 teaspoons poppy seeds

Pinch sea salt

For the salad

5 cups mixed baby greens

2 peaches, pitted and chopped

1 cup fresh blueberries

½ cup toasted unsalted sunflower seeds

2 (6-ounce) cooked chicken breasts, cut into thin strips

1 teaspoon chopped fresh thyme

To make the dressing

1. In a small bowl, whisk the yogurt, honey, balsamic vinegar, extra-virgin olive oil, and poppy seeds until well blended.

2. Season with sea salt and set aside.

To make the salad

1. In a large bowl, toss together the mixed greens, peaches, blueberries, and sunflower seeds until well mixed.

2. Add the dressing and toss to coat.

3. To serve, top the salad with the cooked chicken and sprinkle with thyme.

Cooking tip: Make this salad using leftover roast chicken from dinner. Both dark and white are delicious in it. Dark meat is often juicier than white meat and has a delightful flavor.

PER SERVING Calories: 364; Total Fat: 15g; Saturated Fat: 3g; Carbohydrates: 30g; Fiber: 6g; Protein: 31g

Lebanese Bread Salad (Fattoush)

SERVES 6 TO 8 / PREP TIME: 20 MINUTES

Fattoush *makes a frequent appearance on most Middle Eastern dinner tables. Well-toasted pita chips are the secret to a delicious dish. Serve it immediately after mixing in the pita chips while they are still crisp.*

For the dressing

½ cup freshly squeezed
lemon juice

1 tablespoon extra-virgin olive oil

2 garlic cloves, minced

½ teaspoon sea salt

½ teaspoon freshly
ground black pepper

For the salad

4 cups chopped romaine lettuce

4 Persian cucumbers, chopped

3 ripe tomatoes, chopped

1 scallion, chopped

½ cup pomegranate seeds

½ cup chopped fresh parsley

½ cup fresh mint leaves

2 (8-inch) pita breads, halved,
toasted until golden brown,
broken into bite-size pieces

1 tablespoon ground sumac

To make the dressing

1. In a small bowl, whisk the lemon juice, olive oil, garlic, sea salt, and pepper.

2. Refrigerate for 5 minutes.

To make the salad

1. In a large bowl, combine the romaine lettuce, cucumbers, tomatoes, scallion, pomegranate seeds, parsley, and mint.

2. Add the dressing and pita chips. Sprinkle with sumac and mix lightly to coat with the dressing.

3. Serve immediately.

Ingredient tip: *Sumac is a tangy and lemony spice made from ground berries used in Mediterranean dishes. It is used in salads or to season grilled meat and fish.*

PER SERVING Calories: 142; Total Fat: 3g; Saturated Fat: 1g; Carbohydrates: 26g; Fiber: 3g; Protein: 5g

Basil–Goat Cheese Sandwich

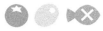

SERVES 4 / PREP TIME: 10 MINUTES / COOK TIME: 25 MINUTES

Roasted red peppers create a striking contrast to the predominantly green toppings in this sandwich. Try orange or yellow peppers instead of red for a variation, keeping in mind as you change the hue, the phytonutrients also change. No matter what color pepper you use, you will benefit from high amounts of calcium, magnesium, potassium, and vitamins A, B, C, and E.

1 head of garlic

Olive oil, for drizzling

4 ounces goat cheese, at room temperature

2 teaspoons chopped fresh basil

Pinch sea salt

Pinch freshly ground black pepper

8 slices whole-wheat or multigrain bread

2 whole roasted red bell peppers, halved, seeded, and cut into thin strips

2 cups shredded spinach

1. Preheat the oven to 350°F.

2. Slice off the top of a head of garlic, just enough to expose the cloves, and then drizzle with olive oil. Place the head in a baking dish, and roast for 20 to 25 minutes in the oven until the cloves are fragrant and soft. Set aside and let cool.

3. In a medium bowl, stir together the goat cheese, basil, 1 teaspoon of the roasted garlic, sea salt, and pepper until very well blended and soft.

4. Toast the bread lightly and spread the goat cheese mixture on 4 slices.

5. Top each slice with one-quarter of the roasted peppers.

6. Heap about ½ cup of spinach on each sandwich, and top each with another slice of toasted bread.

PER SERVING Calories: 322; Total Fat: 11g; Saturated Fat: 7g; Carbohydrates: 35g; Fiber: 11g; Protein: 18g

Summer Vegetable Chicken Wraps

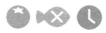

SERVES 4 / PREP TIME: 15 MINUTES

Cucumber adds a pleasing crunch and freshness to the other ingredients, along with a plethora of important nutrients, such as vitamins A, C, and K, as well as magnesium, silicon, beta-carotene, and potassium. Cucumber can help reduce inflammation, blood pressure, and signs of aging while acting as a powerful diuretic.

2 cups chopped cooked chicken

½ English cucumber, diced

½ red bell pepper, diced

½ cup shredded carrot

1 scallion, white and green parts, chopped

¼ cup plain Greek yogurt

1 tablespoon freshly squeezed lemon juice

½ teaspoon chopped fresh thyme

Pinch sea salt

Pinch freshly ground black pepper

4 multigrain tortillas

1. In a medium bowl, mix the chicken, cucumber, red bell pepper, carrot, scallion, yogurt, lemon juice, thyme, sea salt, and pepper until well mixed.

2. Spoon one-quarter of the chicken mixture into the middle of a tortilla. Fold the opposite ends of the tortilla over the filling and then roll the tortilla from the side to create a snug pocket. Repeat with the remaining ingredients.

3. Serve 1 wrap per person.

Substitution tip: *If you want a fresh-tasting treat, use whole romaine lettuce or Boston lettuce leaves instead of tortillas to wrap your sandwich. Lettuce wraps, very popular in many Asian countries, are often served as street food.*

PER SERVING Calories: 278; Total Fat: 7g; Saturated Fat: 2g; Carbohydrates: 28g; Fiber: 6g; Protein: 27g

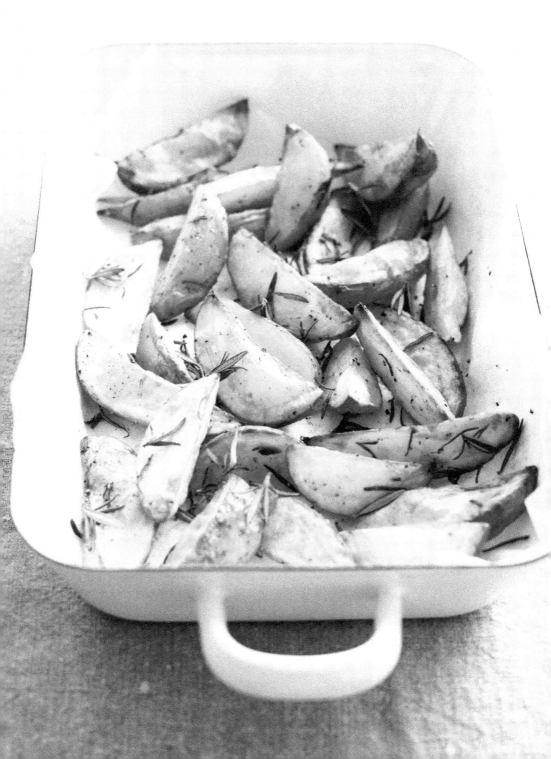

CHAPTER 6

Sides & Snacks

Herb-Roasted Baby Potatoes

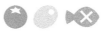

SERVES 4 / PREP TIME: 10 MINUTES / COOK TIME: 35 MINUTES

Roasted potatoes with crispy edges and a hint of herbs rank as a favorite side dish for most people. Paprika helps create a golden color and, if you use the smoked spice, it adds an incredible taste as well. Made from dried red peppers, paprika is used in Hungarian and Spanish cuisines.

2 pounds new yellow or red potatoes, scrubbed and cut into wedges

2 tablespoons extra-virgin olive oil

2 teaspoons chopped fresh rosemary

1 teaspoon garlic powder

1 teaspoon sweet paprika, or smoked paprika

½ teaspoon sea salt

½ teaspoon freshly ground black pepper

1. Preheat the oven to 400ºF.
2. Line a baking sheet with aluminum foil and set aside.
3. In a large bowl, toss together the potatoes, olive oil, rosemary, garlic powder, paprika, sea salt, and pepper.
4. Spread the potatoes in a single layer on the baking sheet. Bake for about 35 minutes or until golden brown and tender.
5. Serve.

Cooking tip: If you want to save time, blanch your potatoes whole, chill them, and then cut them into wedges just before tossing with the oil and seasonings. This can cut baking time by about 20 minutes.

PER SERVING Calories: 225; Total Fat: 7g; Saturated Fat: 1g; Carbohydrates: 37g; Fiber: 4g; Protein: 5g

Fennel Wild Rice

SERVES 6 / PREP TIME: 10 MINUTES / COOK TIME: 11 MINUTES

Fennel is an undeniably handsome vegetable, like a fat bunch of celery with feathery fronds. Fennel tastes more like licorice than celery, and the flavor mellows beautifully when cooked. This vegetable supports a healthy heart and digestion while helping cut the risk of cancer because it is very high in potassium, iron, B vitamins, and vitamin C.

1 tablespoon extra-virgin olive oil

1 cup diced fennel

½ red bell pepper, finely diced

½ cup chopped sweet onion

2 cups cooked wild rice

1 tablespoon chopped fresh parsley

Sea salt

Freshly ground black pepper

1. In a large skillet over medium-high heat, heat the olive oil.

2. Add the fennel, red bell pepper, and onion. Sauté for about 6 minutes, or until tender.

3. Stir in the wild rice. Cook for about 5 minutes until heated through.

4. Add the parsley, and season with sea salt and pepper.

Ingredient tip: Wild rice is not really rice but an aquatic grass that grows in lakes and rivers in parts of Minnesota and Canada. Cooked wild rice can be kept refrigerated in a covered container for up to 4 days.

PER SERVING Calories: 222; Total Fat: 3g; Saturated Fat: 0g; Carbohydrates: 43g; Fiber: 4g; Protein: 8g

Scalloped Tomatoes

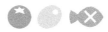

SERVES 4 / PREP TIME: 15 MINUTES / COOK TIME: 40 MINUTES

The term scalloped *is often thought to mean something in a creamy cheesy sauce, but it can also mean baked, as is the case with this delectable side. The bread chunks soak up the liquid from the tomatoes, creating a sauce-like texture. Crusty French bread can be used in place of whole-wheat if you prefer.*

1 tablespoon extra-virgin
  olive oil, divided

2 slices whole-wheat bread,
  cut into ½-inch cubes

1 tablespoon minced garlic

2¼ pounds tomatoes,
  cut into eighths

Sea salt

Freshly ground black pepper

¼ cup chopped fresh basil

2 tablespoons shredded
  Asiago cheese

1. Preheat the oven to 350°F.

2. Lightly grease an 8-by-8-inch baking dish with ½ teaspoon of olive oil and set aside.

3. In a large skillet over medium-high heat, heat the remaining 2½ teaspoons of olive oil.

4. Add the bread cubes and sauté for about 4 minutes until they're golden brown on all sides.

5. Add the garlic to the skillet and sauté for 2 minutes.

6. Stir in the tomatoes and sauté for 2 minutes.

7. Remove the skillet from the heat and season the tomato mixture with sea salt and pepper.

8. Stir in the basil and transfer the mixture to the prepared dish.

9. Sprinkle the Asiago cheese evenly on top and bake for 30 minutes.

Ingredient tip: *Basil is usually sold in rather large bunches, creating a surplus when you don't need it all for a recipe. Freeze any extra: Put whole basil stems on a baking sheet in the freezer. Once completely frozen, transfer the herbs to storage containers. Store the containers in the freezer for up to 1 month.*

PER SERVING Calories: 127; Total Fat: 6g; Saturated Fat: 1g; Carbohydrates: 16g; Fiber: 4g; Protein: 5g

Brussels Sprouts with Pistachios

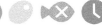

SERVES 4 / PREP TIME: 15 MINUTES / COOK TIME: 15 MINUTES

Brussels sprouts are often thought of in the same terms as cabbage—soggy peasant food with an unpleasant pungent odor while cooking. Brussels sprouts are actually tender and delicious when prepared well. The best and healthiest method of cooking Brussels sprouts is roasting because the sulforaphane, a cancer-fighting chemical in this vegetable, is destroyed when boiled. Try adding cashews, hazelnuts, or almonds to this dish instead of pistachios.

1 pound Brussels sprouts, tough bottoms trimmed, halved lengthwise

4 shallots, peeled and quartered

1 tablespoon extra-virgin olive oil

Sea salt

Freshly ground black pepper

½ cup chopped roasted pistachios

Zest of ½ lemon

Juice of ½ lemon

1. Preheat the oven to 400°F.

2. Line a baking sheet with aluminum foil and set aside.

3. In a large bowl, toss the Brussels sprouts and shallots with the olive oil until well coated.

4. Season with sea salt and pepper, and then spread the vegetables evenly on the sheet.

5. Bake for 15 minutes, or until tender and lightly caramelized.

6. Remove from the oven and transfer to a serving bowl.

7. Toss with the pistachios, lemon zest, and lemon juice. Serve warm.

Substitution tip: Nuts can be omitted if you need to be careful about an allergy. Brussels sprouts with a hint of lemon are still delicious.

PER SERVING Calories: 126; Total Fat: 7g; Saturated Fat: 1g; Carbohydrates: 14g; Fiber: 5g; Protein: 6g

Roasted Parmesan Broccoli

SERVES 4 / PREP TIME: 10 MINUTES / COOK TIME: 10 MINUTES

One of the criticisms of broccoli in side dishes is that it is limp or mushy from being boiled too long. Roasting the florets with a sprinkling of rich Parmesan cheese creates a crisp-tender texture and smoky flavor that will silence any broccoli critics. Broccoli is very low on the glycemic index and is an excellent source of fiber, chromium, and vitamins K, C, and A.

2 heads broccoli, cut into small florets

2 tablespoons extra-virgin olive oil, plus more for greasing the baking sheet

2 teaspoons minced garlic

Zest of 1 lemon

Juice of 1 lemon

Pinch sea salt

½ cup grated Parmesan cheese

1. Preheat the oven to 400ºF.
2. Lightly grease a baking sheet with olive oil and set aside.
3. In a large bowl, toss the broccoli with the 2 tablespoons of olive oil, garlic, lemon zest, lemon juice, and sea salt.
4. Spread the mixture on the baking sheet in a single layer and sprinkle with the Parmesan cheese.
5. Bake for about 10 minutes, or until tender. Transfer the broccoli to a serving dish and serve.

Cooking tip: Leave the florets on the stalk and don't wash broccoli until you are ready to cook it. Cutting this vegetable prematurely diminishes its vitamin C levels. For best results, simply refrigerate broccoli in a sealed plastic bag for up to 1 week.

PER SERVING Calories: 154; Total Fat: 11g; Saturated Fat: 3g; Carbohydrates: 10g; Fiber: 4; Protein: 9g

Mashed Celeriac

SERVES 4 / PREP TIME: 10 MINUTES / COOK TIME: 20 MINUTES

You might think you have stumbled into the gardening section of the local supermarket when you look at a pile of lumpy, hairy celeriac. This unusual, bulbous root has a fresh celery flavor and interesting firm texture that mashes as fluffy as potatoes. You can vary this tasty side dish to create interesting combinations by adding sweet potato, squash, and parsnip.

2 celeriac (celery root), washed, peeled, and diced

2 teaspoons extra-virgin olive oil

1 tablespoon honey

½ teaspoon ground nutmeg

Sea salt

Freshly ground black pepper

1. Preheat the oven to 400°F.

2. Line a baking sheet with aluminum foil and set aside.

3. In a large bowl, toss together the celeriac and olive oil. Spread the celeriac pieces evenly on the baking sheet, and roast for about 20 minutes until very tender and lightly caramelized. Transfer to a large bowl.

4. Add the honey and nutmeg. Use a potato masher to mash the ingredients until fluffy.

5. Season with sea salt and pepper before serving.

Ingredient tip: Nutmeg has a sweet, warm taste, which can be bitter if the spice is too old or stored in direct sunlight. Buy whole nutmeg and use a micro grater for the most intense flavor and best quality.

PER SERVING Calories: 136; Total Fat: 3g; Saturated Fat: 1g; Carbohydrates: 26g; Fiber: 4g; Protein: 4g

Lebanese Rice Pilaf

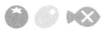

SERVES 4 / PREP TIME: 5 MINUTES / COOK TIME: 35 MINUTES

A staple in Middle Eastern cuisine, Lebanese rice pilaf is made with vermicelli noodles toasted in olive oil before being added to the rice. Vermicelli is long, slender pasta, thinner than spaghetti.

½ cup vermicelli, broken in 2 inch pieces

1 tablespoon extra-virgin olive oil

1 cup uncooked long-grain rice

2 cups water

1 teaspoon sea salt

1. In a saucepan over medium heat, cook the vermicelli with the olive oil for about 5 minutes until golden brown.

2. Rinse the rice in cold water, drain, and add to the vermicelli. Sauté for 2 minutes.

3. Add the water and sea salt. Cover and cook for 20 minutes.

4. Reduce the heat to low and simmer for 5 minutes more, or until the rice and vermicelli are tender.

Ingredient tip: Toasted vermicelli can be used in many ways. After toasting the vermicelli with olive oil, you can add to it to stir-fries and salads for some texture without bulk.

PER SERVING Calories: 251; Total Fat: 4g; Saturated Fat: 1g; Carbohydrates: 47g; Fiber: 1g; Protein: 5g

Chili Kale Chips

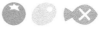

SERVES 4 / PREP TIME: 10 MINUTES / COOK TIME: 25 MINUTES

Kale chips are a current sensation. Use this recipe as a base to try any type of herb or spice you like until you hit on a winning taste combination. Chili powder comes in different types, from smoky chipotle to throat-searing hot, depending on the chile pepper used. The substance that creates the heat is called capsaicin, which as an ointment, is an effective treatment for osteoarthritis pain.

3 cups kale, stemmed, thoroughly washed, and torn into 2-inch pieces

1 tablespoon extra-virgin olive oil

½ teaspoon chili powder

¼ teaspoon sea salt

1. Preheat the oven to 300°F.

2. Line 2 baking sheets with parchment paper and set aside.

3. Dry the kale completely and transfer to a large bowl. Add the olive oil and toss together, making sure that each leaf is coated.

4. Season the kale with chili powder and sea salt, tossing again to coat evenly. Divide the kale between the baking sheets and spread it into a single layer.

5. Bake for about 25 minutes until dry and crispy, rotating the sheets halfway through.

6. Cool the chips for 5 minutes before serving.

Cooking tip: Take extra time to dry each piece of kale thoroughly before tossing with the olive oil or your chips won't be uniformly crisp. Water repels the oil, creating soggy spots on the kale leaves.

PER SERVING Calories: 56; Total Fat: 4g; Saturated Fat: 1g; Carbohydrates: 5g; Fiber: 1g; Protein: 2g

Hummus

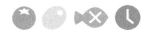

SERVES 6 / PREP TIME: 5 MINUTES

Hummus is much more popular throughout America today than it ever was in the past. It is a tasty and healthy alternative to most other dips and spreads, and is a delightful and common side dish in Mediterranean cuisines.

1 (16-ounce) can chickpeas, or garbanzo beans, drained

½ cup freshly squeezed lemon juice

1½ tablespoons tahini

3 garlic cloves, crushed

1 tablespoon extra-virgin olive oil

1 teaspoon sea salt

1. In a blender or food processor, combine the chickpeas, lemon juice, tahini, garlic, olive oil, and sea salt. Blend for 3 to 5 minutes on low until thoroughly mixed and smooth. The texture should be soft and fluffy.

2. For best results, refrigerate for 1 hour before serving with warm pita bread or cut vegetables, as desired.

Cooking tip: You can also add your favorite seasoning or spices to enhance the flavor of this hummus. Try cumin, coriander, paprika, or roasted red peppers.

PER SERVING Calories: 187; Total Fat: 7g; Saturated Fat: 1g; Carbohydrates: 25g; Fiber: 7g; Protein: 8g

Herbed Yogurt Dip

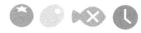

SERVES 4 / PREP TIME: 10 MINUTES

Everyone should have a good no-fail dip when company drops by unexpectedly and you need something tasty to serve. Any combination of fresh herbs works, so you can throw in basil, oregano, summer savory, rosemary, marjoram, and even a sprinkling of sage. If you have any left over, thin it with a bit of milk or water and drizzle it over fresh greens for a simple salad dressing.

1 cup plain Greek yogurt

Zest of ½ lemon

Juice of ½ lemon

1 tablespoon finely chopped fresh chives

2 teaspoons chopped fresh dill

2 teaspoons chopped fresh thyme

1 teaspoon chopped fresh parsley

½ teaspoon minced garlic

Pinch sea salt

1. In a medium bowl, stir together the yogurt, lemon zest, lemon juice, chives, dill, thyme, parsley, and garlic until very well blended.

2. Season with the sea salt and transfer to a sealed container.

3. Keep refrigerated for up to 2 weeks.

Cooking tip: If you have ever seen dill for sale in the grocery store you might be envisioning a huge bunch of stems that would be more appropriate for a vase on the kitchen table. If you need only a small bit of this herb, look for tubes of puréed dill in the produce section. Simply squeeze out the required quantity and refrigerate the rest.

PER SERVING Calories: 59; Total Fat: 4g; Saturated Fat: 2g; Carbohydrates: 5g; Fiber: 4g; Protein: 2g

Seed and Nut Snack Bars

MAKES 8 BARS / PREP TIME: 20 MINUTES, PLUS 4 HOURS FREEZING

Purchased granola bars seem like a healthy option, but in most cases, they are simply cookies in disguise with a ton of sugar and saturated fat. Once you try these homemade seed and nut bars, you will be hooked on the delightful flavor and complete lack of additives. This recipe can be altered with other dried fruits, nuts, and seeds in place of ones you don't like or don't have on hand.

½ cup Medjool dates

½ cup almonds

¼ cup sunflower seeds

¼ cup pecans

1 cup dried cranberries

2 tablespoons sesame seeds

1 tablespoon flaxseed

1 tablespoon honey

1. Cut a piece of parchment paper to fit the bottom of an 8-by-8-inch baking dish and set the lined dish aside.

2. In a food processor, pulse the dates, almonds, sunflower seeds, and pecans until they are very finely chopped.

3. Add the cranberries, sesame seeds, flaxseed, and honey, and pulse until the mixture starts to form a ball.

4. Press the mixture very firmly into the prepared baking dish with lightly greased fingers to prevent sticking.

5. Cover with plastic wrap and place the baking dish in the refrigerator for 4 hours to firm.

6. Cut into 8 bars and store them in a sealed container for up to 2 weeks.

Cooking tip: *Make a double or triple batch of bars for a quick grab-and-go snack or breakfast. These bars, wrapped individually, also freeze beautifully for at least 3 months.*

PER SERVING Calories: 103; Total Fat: 6g; Saturated Fat: 1g; Carbohydrates: 10g; Fiber: 3g; Protein: 3g

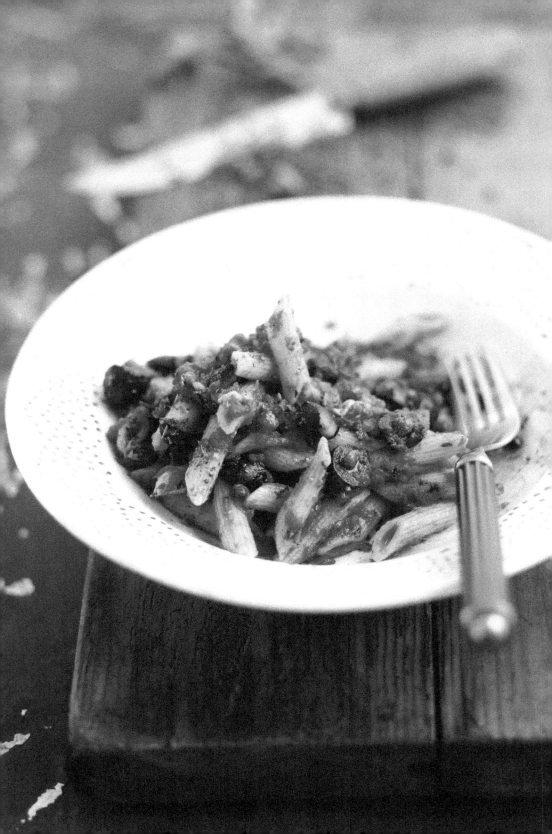

CHAPTER 7

Pizza & Pasta

Southwest Pizza

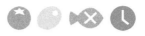

SERVES 4 / PREP TIME: 15 MINUTES / COOK TIME: 10 MINUTES

Pita breads make handy crusts for personal-size pizzas, and they crisp beautifully to mimic a thin pizza crust. The Southwest flavor of this dish is created with fiery jalapeños, silky mashed beans, peppers, feta cheese, and a generous scattering of cilantro. Try grilling the pita breads on a low-heat barbecue for an added smoky flavor.

4 (6-inch) whole-wheat pita breads

1 tablespoon extra-virgin olive oil

2 cups canned sodium-free white navy beans, drained and rinsed

1 scallion, white and green parts, finely chopped

1 jalapeño pepper, seeded and finely chopped

1 teaspoon ground cumin

1 tomato, diced

1 yellow bell pepper, thinly sliced

½ cup crumbled feta cheese

4 teaspoons chopped fresh cilantro

1. Preheat the oven to 400°F.

2. Place the pita breads on a baking sheet and lightly brush both sides with olive oil. Bake for about 5 minutes until golden brown and crispy, turning once.

3. In a medium bowl, mash together the beans, scallion, jalapeño, and cumin to form a chunky paste.

4. Evenly divide the bean mixture among the toasted pita breads, spreading it to the edges.

5. Top each with tomato, yellow bell pepper, and feta cheese.

6. Bake the pizzas for about 3 minutes until the cheese is slightly melted.

7. Sprinkle with cilantro and serve.

Cooking tip: *Serve this pizza with homemade salsa or pico de gallo and a spoonful of plain Greek yogurt to complete the Southwest touch.*

PER SERVING Calories: 387; Total Fat: 9g; Saturated Fat: 3g; Carbohydrates: 64g; Fiber: 16g; Protein: 17g

Caramelized Onion and Fennel Pizza

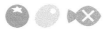

SERVES 4 / PREP TIME: 15 MINUTES / COOK TIME: 35 MINUTES

Producing perfectly caramelized onions is a skill coveted by professional chefs everywhere. This process takes time, patience, and the ability to know when the onions are sweet and golden rather than slightly scorched and bitter. If you want to speed up the timing a little, add ¼ teaspoon baking soda per whole onion and you will have slightly soft but caramelized, onions in as little as 10 minutes.

1 (10-inch) pizza crust, homemade or premade

1 tablespoon extra-virgin olive oil, divided

4 cups sliced sweet onions

4 cups thinly sliced fennel

1 teaspoon chopped fresh oregano

1 teaspoon dried thyme

¼ teaspoon freshly ground black pepper

¼ teaspoon sea salt

½ cup grated Parmesan cheese

1. Preheat the oven to 450°F.

2. Place the pizza crust on a baking sheet and lightly brush the edges with 1 teaspoon of olive oil.

3. In a large skillet over medium-high heat, heat the remaining 2 teaspoons of olive oil.

4. Add the onions, fennel, oregano, thyme, pepper, and sea salt. Sauté for about 25 minutes, stirring frequently until the vegetables are caramelized and tender.

5. Spread the vegetables over the crust to about ½ inch from the edge.

6. Sprinkle the vegetables with Parmesan cheese.

7. Bake for 10 to 12 minutes, or until the crust is crisp and golden.

8. Cut the pizza into 8 pieces and serve 2 per person.

Ingredient tip: Purchase fennel that has no flowering buds in the fronds. These pretty flowers mean the vegetable is past its prime and it can be bitter.

PER SERVING Calories: 225; Total Fat: 8g; Saturated Fat: 3g; Carbohydrates: 33g; Fiber: 6g; Protein: 10g

Shrimp and Mango Pizza

SERVES 4 / PREP TIME: 15 MINUTES / COOK TIME: 20 MINUTES

Cilantro adds a bright splash of green to this pizza—along with many vitamins and minerals. This herb is a staple addition to Asian and Latino cooking, because it combines well with assertive flavors. Cilantro is an excellent source of vitamins A, C, and K, as well as iron and calcium.

1 tablespoon extra-virgin olive oil

1 teaspoon minced garlic

½ teaspoon grated peeled fresh ginger

½ pound (21 to 25 count) shrimp, shelled and deveined

4 (6-inch) whole-wheat pita breads, or multigrain pita breads

Juice of 1 lime

1 mango, peeled, pitted, and diced

1 scallion, white and green parts, chopped

½ jalapeño pepper, seeded and minced

Pinch sea salt

1 tablespoon chopped fresh cilantro

1. Preheat the oven to 375ºF.

2. In a large skillet over medium-high heat, heat the olive oil.

3. Add the garlic and ginger and sauté for about 2 minutes until tender.

4. Add the shrimp. Sauté for about 4 minutes, until pink and opaque. Transfer the shrimp to a bowl and cool for 15 minutes.

5. Place the pita breads on a baking sheet and bake for about 10 minutes, turning once, until crisp and golden.

6. While the pita is toasting, add the lime juice, mango, scallion, jalapeño, and sea salt to the shrimp and toss to mix.

7. Spread the shrimp mixture on the toasted pitas and garnish with cilantro.

Substitution tip: *Chopped chicken or diced bell peppers and tomatoes can replace the shrimp if a seafood-free or vegetarian version is required.*

PER SERVING Calories: 307; Total Fat: 6g; Saturated Fat: 1g; Carbohydrates: 46g; Fiber: 6g; Protein: 20g

Spinach Chicken Pizza

SERVES 4 / PREP TIME: 15 MINUTES / COOK TIME: 15 MINUTES

Premade pizza dough is available in most grocery stores, either in the bakery section or frozen food aisle, and you can often find plain and whole-wheat versions. These convenience products contain the same ingredients you would put in your own dough, so don't be afraid to use them. You can even pick up a prebaked pizza crust if you enjoy a thicker more bread-like version.

1 (9-inch) pizza crust, homemade or premade

½ teaspoon extra-virgin olive oil

1 cup chopped tomato

¼ teaspoon red pepper flakes

2 cups chopped blanched fresh spinach

1 tablespoon chopped fresh basil

1 cup chopped cooked chicken breast

1 cup shredded Asiago cheese

1. Preheat the oven to 400°F.

2. Prepare the pizza dough according to your recipe or package instructions and roll it out to form a 9-inch crust. Transfer the crust to a baking sheet, and brush the edges lightly with olive oil.

3. Spread the tomato and red pepper flakes over the pizza leaving the oiled crust bare.

4. Arrange the spinach and basil over the tomato, and scatter the chopped chicken on the spinach. Top with the Asiago cheese.

5. Bake the pizza for about 15 minutes until the crust is crispy and the cheese is melted.

Ingredient tip: *Do not skip the blanching step for the spinach, because this green can dry out and burn when exposed to a high-heat oven. Squeeze out as much water as possible from the spinach after cooking it so the pizza won't be mushy.*

PER SERVING Calories: 255; Total Fat: 11g; Saturated Fat: 5g; Carbohydrates: 17g; Fiber: 2g; Protein: 23g

Pesto Veggie Pizza

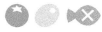

SERVES 4 / PREP TIME: 25 MINUTES / COOK TIME: 20 MINUTES

Pizza is often portrayed in movies, TV shows, and ads as an artery-clogging, calorie-laden indulgence with no place in a healthy diet. Although likely true for purchased pizzas, creating one at home lets you control what goes on it. This flavorful pizza is heaped with delicious—and healthy—vegetables and cheese.

Flour, for dusting

1 (10-inch) pizza crust, homemade or premade

½ cup sun-dried tomato pesto

1 cup sliced button mushrooms

1 red bell pepper, chopped

½ cup sliced zucchini

½ cup thinly sliced red onion, divided

½ cup sliced black olives

½ cup grated Parmesan cheese

1. Preheat the oven to 400°F.

2. Line a baking sheet with parchment paper and set aside.

3. Dust your work surface with flour, and roll out the pizza dough so it forms a 10-inch circle. Transfer the pizza dough to the prepared baking sheet.

4. Spread the pesto over the dough to 1 inch from the edge.

5. Arrange the mushrooms, red bell pepper, zucchini, onion, and olives on the pizza and top with the Parmesan cheese.

6. Bake for about 20 minutes until golden and crispy, and the cheese melts.

Substitution tip: Instead of sun-dried tomato pesto, try basil or herb pesto—either homemade or a good-quality purchased brand. Use the same amount as the sun-dried tomato pesto.

PER SERVING Calories: 210; Total Fat: 9g; Saturated Fat: 3g; Carbohydrates: 25g; Fiber: 4g; Protein: 9g

Macaroni with Milk
(Macaroni bil-Halib)

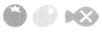

SERVES 10 TO 12 / PREP TIME: 10 MINUTES / COOK TIME: 35 TO 45 MINUTES

This delicious vegetarian dish is common in Lebanon. It always brings me back to my childhood—coming home to a simple bowl of mac and cheese, but without the cheese. You can use any type of pasta you like. I prefer angel hair. If you like this to be a little thick, use a smaller baking dish, 8-by-11 inches, but if you like it thinner, use a 9-by-13-inch baking dish.

1 tablespoon extra-virgin olive oil

1 pound spaghetti

4 cups milk

3 large eggs, well beaten

1 tablespoon ground allspice

1 teaspoon sea salt

¼ teaspoon pure vanilla extract

¼ cup plain bread crumbs

1. Preheat the oven to 350°F.

2. Grease a 9-by-13-inch baking dish with olive oil and set aside.

3. Cook the spaghetti according to the package directions. Rinse in cold water, drain, and place in the prepared dish.

4. In a food processor, combine the milk, eggs, allspice, sea salt, and vanilla. Process until blended and then pour the mixture over the spaghetti.

5. Top with the bread crumbs and bake for 35 to 45 minutes, or until golden brown and set.

Cooking tip: For even more flavor, sprinkle some of your favorite cheese over the pasta before adding the bread crumbs. Shredded mozzarella is a great choice.

PER SERVING Calories: 224; Total Fat: 7g; Saturated Fat: 3g; Carbohydrates: 32g; Fiber: 0g; Protein: 10g

Linguine with Cherry Tomatoes

SERVES 4 / PREP TIME: 10 MINUTES / COOK TIME: 15 MINUTES

Cherry tomatoes are nature's perfect snack, the perfect size to pop in your mouth—preferably picked fresh and warmed from the sun. This dish depends on the intense, sweet flavor of ripe cherry tomatoes, so make sure you source the ripest possible. Combine yellow and red tomatoes for an interesting presentation, or use assorted heirloom fruit, if available.

2 pounds cherry tomatoes

3 tablespoons extra-virgin olive oil

2 tablespoons balsamic vinegar

2 teaspoons minced garlic

Pinch freshly ground black pepper

¾ pound whole-wheat linguine pasta

1 tablespoon chopped fresh oregano

¼ cup crumbled feta cheese

1. Preheat the oven to 350ºF.

2. Line a baking sheet with parchment paper and set aside.

3. In a large bowl, toss the cherry tomatoes with 2 tablespoons of olive oil, the balsamic vinegar, garlic, and pepper until well coated. Spread the tomatoes evenly on the prepared sheet and roast for about 15 minutes until they are softened and burst open.

4. While the tomatoes roast, cook the pasta according to package directions. Drain and transfer to a large bowl.

5. Toss the pasta with the remaining 1 tablespoon of olive oil.

6. Add the roasted tomatoes, taking care to get all the juices and bits from the baking sheet. Toss to combine.

7. To serve, top with the oregano and feta cheese.

Substitution tip: *Chopped cooked chicken or lean cooked turkey sausage would be fabulous additions if having a vegetarian dish isn't important. Add the proteins to the bowl with the rest of the ingredients and toss to combine.*

PER SERVING Calories: 397; Total Fat: 15g; Saturated Fat: 3g; Carbohydrates: 55g; Fiber: 6g; Protein: 13g

Linguine with Tomato Clam Sauce

SERVES 4 / PREP TIME: 10 MINUTES / COOK TIME: 10 MINUTES

Garlic infuses every delectable bite of this complex sauce. Garlic is a health powerhouse with more than 70 phytochemicals, as well as calcium, selenium, fiber, manganese, and vitamin B_1. This allium can help reduce the risk of cancer, lower blood pressure, and even fight the common cold.

1 pound linguine

Pinch sea salt

1 teaspoon extra-virgin olive oil

1 tablespoon minced garlic

1 teaspoon chopped fresh thyme

½ teaspoon red pepper flakes

1 (15-ounce) can sodium-free diced tomatoes, drained

1 (15-ounce) can whole baby clams, with their juice

Sea salt

Freshly ground black pepper

2 tablespoons chopped fresh parsley

1. Cook the linguine according to the package directions.

2. While the linguine cooks, heat the olive oil in a large skillet over medium heat.

3. Add the garlic, thyme, and red pepper flakes. Sauté for about 3 minutes until softened.

4. Stir in the tomatoes and clams. Bring the sauce to a boil, reduce the heat to low, and simmer for 5 minutes.

5. Season with sea salt and pepper.

6. Drain the cooked pasta and toss it with the sauce.

7. Garnish with the parsley and serve.

PER SERVING Calories: 394; Total Fat: 5g; Saturated Fat: 0g; Carbohydrates: 66g; Fiber: 7g; Protein: 23g

Angel Hair with Asparagus-Kale Pesto

SERVES 6 / PREP TIME: 10 MINUTES / COOK TIME: 10 MINUTES

Cooking angel hair pasta asks you to be a pro! It takes your full attention. You must watch carefully and remove it from the water before it overcooks to put together this delicate-looking and tasting meal because the angel hair seems to cradle the pesto. You can certainly use spaghetti, if you prefer.

¾ pound asparagus, woody ends removed, and coarsely chopped

¼ pound kale, thoroughly washed

½ cup grated Asiago cheese

¼ cup fresh basil

¼ cup extra-virgin olive oil

Juice of 1 lemon

Sea salt

Freshly ground black pepper

1 pound angel hair pasta

Zest of 1 lemon

1. In a food processor, pulse the asparagus and kale until very finely chopped.
2. Add the Asiago cheese, basil, olive oil, and lemon juice and pulse to form a smooth pesto.
3. Season with sea salt and pepper and set aside.
4. Cook the pasta al dente according to the package directions. Drain and transfer to a large bowl.
5. Add the pesto, tossing well to coat.
6. Sprinkle with lemon zest and serve.

Cooking tip: You can make the asparagus pesto up to 3 days ahead. Keep it refrigerated until you need it.

PER SERVING Calories: 283; Total Fat: 12g; Saturated Fat: 2g; Carbohydrates: 33g; Fiber: 2g; Protein: 10g

Spicy Pasta Puttanesca

SERVES 4 / PREP TIME: 10 MINUTES / COOK TIME: 20 MINUTES

Puttanesca *is probably the most colorful name of a sauce; it means "harlot style." The salty, rich flavor of the dish is created by the anchovies, olives, and capers. If you dislike anchovies, leave them out for the Neapolitan version of this recipe. You might want to try the sauce "as is," though, because this dish is exceptional.*

2 teaspoons extra-virgin olive oil

½ sweet onion, finely chopped

2 teaspoons minced garlic

1 (28-ounce) can sodium-free diced tomatoes

½ cup chopped anchovies

2 teaspoons chopped fresh oregano

2 teaspoons chopped fresh basil

½ teaspoon red pepper flakes

½ cup quartered Kalamata olives

¼ cup sodium-free chicken broth

1 tablespoon capers, drained and rinsed

Juice of 1 lemon

4 cups cooked whole-grain penne

1. In a large saucepan over medium heat, heat the olive oil.

2. Add the onion and garlic, and sauté for about 3 minutes until softened.

3. Stir in the tomatoes, anchovies, oregano, basil, and red pepper flakes. Bring the sauce to a boil and reduce the heat to low. Simmer for 15 minutes, stirring occasionally.

4. Stir in the olives, chicken broth, capers, and lemon juice.

5. Cook the pasta according to the package directions and serve topped with the sauce.

Ingredient tip: *Do not mistake sardines for anchovies, although they are both small, silvery fish sold in cans. Anchovies are usually salted in brine and matured to create a distinctive, rich taste.*

PER SERVING Calories: 303; Total Fat: 6g; Saturated Fat: 0g; Carbohydrates: 54g; Fiber: 9g; Protein: 9g

Roasted Vegetarian Lasagna

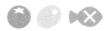

SERVES 6 / PREP TIME: 25 MINUTES / COOK TIME: 50 MINUTES

There are very few vegetables that don't benefit from roasting until lightly caramelized and tender. The ones in this casserole are just a guide for quantities because you can substitute whatever you desire with the same outstanding results. Fennel, asparagus, green beans, cauliflower, and sweet bell peppers are other appealing options.

1 eggplant, thickly sliced

2 zucchini, sliced lengthwise

1 yellow squash, sliced lengthwise

1 sweet onion, thickly sliced

2 tablespoons extra-virgin olive oil

1 (28-ounce) can sodium-free diced tomatoes

1 cup quartered, canned, water-packed artichoke hearts, drained

2 teaspoons minced garlic

2 teaspoons chopped fresh basil

2 teaspoons chopped fresh oregano

Pinch red pepper flakes

12 no-boil whole-grain lasagna noodles

¾ cup grated Asiago cheese

1. Preheat the oven to 400°F.

2. Line a baking sheet with aluminum foil and set aside.

3. In a large bowl, toss together the eggplant, zucchini, yellow squash, onion, and olive oil to coat.

4. Arrange the vegetables on the prepared sheet and roast for about 20 minutes, or until tender and lightly caramelized.

5. Chop the roasted vegetables well and transfer them to a large bowl.

6. Stir in the tomatoes, artichoke hearts, garlic, basil, oregano, and red pepper flakes.

7. Spoon one-quarter of the vegetable mixture into the bottom of a deep 9-by-13-inch baking dish.

8. Arrange 4 lasagna noodles over the sauce.

9. Repeat, alternating sauce and noodles, ending with sauce.

10. Sprinkle the Asiago cheese evenly over the top. Bake for about 30 minutes until bubbly and hot.

11. Remove from the oven and cool for 15 minutes before serving.

Substitution tip: If having a vegetarian meal is not a requirement, lean ground beef (92%) or ground chicken can be added to the roasted vegetable sauce for a more robust meal. Brown the ground meat in a skillet and add it to the finished sauce before assembling the lasagna.

PER SERVING Calories: 386; Total Fat: 11g; Saturated Fat: 3g; Carbohydrates: 59g; Fiber: 12g; Protein: 15g

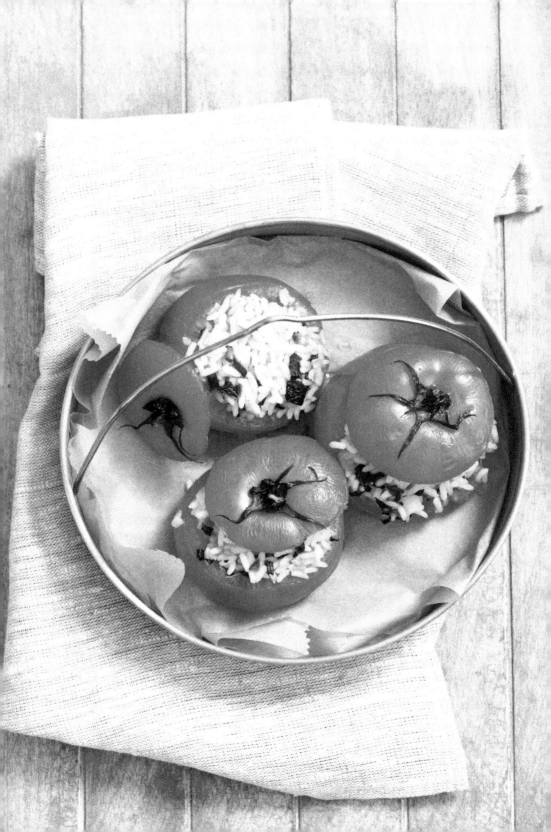

CHAPTER 8

Vegetarian

Butternut Squash and White Bean Pilaf

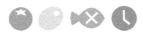

SERVES 6 / PREP TIME: 10 MINUTES / COOK TIME: 20 MINUTES

Pilaf is often a hot dish of rice cooked in a seasoned broth, but this pilaf is served at room temperature and the rice is flavored with a spiced dressing. If you prefer a hotter meal, skip the chilling step for the roasted vegetables, and toss them right out of the oven with the other ingredients.

For the dressing

¼ cup extra-virgin olive oil

3 tablespoons honey

2 tablespoons freshly
  squeezed lemon juice

¼ teaspoon ground cumin

Pinch ground cinnamon

Pinch sea salt

Pinch freshly ground
  black pepper

For the salad

2 large parsnips, peeled and diced

1 small butternut squash,
  peeled and diced

1 large carrot, peeled and diced

1 tablespoon extra-virgin olive oil

1 cup cooked sodium-free white
  navy beans, drained and rinsed

1 cup cooked brown rice

1 scallion, white and green
  parts, thinly sliced diagonally

To make the dressing

In a small bowl, whisk the olive oil, honey, lemon juice, cumin, cinnamon, sea salt, and pepper. Set aside.

To make the salad

1. Preheat the oven to 375ºF.

2. Line a baking sheet with aluminum foil and set aside.

3. In a large bowl, toss together the parsnips, squash, carrot, and olive oil. Spread the vegetables on the prepared sheet and bake for about 20 minutes until caramelized and soft.

4. Remove from the oven and let cool, and then transfer to a large bowl.

5. Add the white beans, brown rice, scallion, and dressing to the bowl. Toss to coat.

Ingredient tip: Scallions are also called green onions, even though they are immature lily bulbs, not onions. Scallions are best when they have vibrant green stalks and clean-looking white bulbs with no wet layers.

PER SERVING Calories: 290; Total Fat: 12g; Saturated Fat: 2g; Carbohydrates: 46g; Fiber: 9g; Protein: 8g

Lentil Sesame Patties

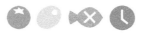

SERVES 4 / PREP TIME: 20 MINUTES, PLUS 1 HOUR CHILLING / COOK TIME: 5 MINUTES

Fresh ginger adds heat and a great deal of flavor to these golden patties. Fresh ginger is the rhizome of the ginger plant and is characterized by a bulbous appearance and brown skin. Ginger helps ease digestive problems, which explains why mothers everywhere pour ginger ale for upset tummies. Fresh ginger has a more complex, but milder, flavor than ground ginger, so if you use the spice instead, use only one teaspoon.

2 cups cooked red lentils

2 large eggs, beaten

¼ cup whole-wheat bread crumbs, plus more as needed

¼ cup chopped sweet onion

2 teaspoons minced garlic

2 teaspoons grated peeled fresh ginger

¾ cup sesame seeds

2 tablespoons extra-virgin olive oil

1. In a large bowl, mash together the red lentils, eggs, bread crumbs, onion, garlic, and ginger until well mixed and the ingredients hold together when pressed. Add more bread crumbs or a little water, as needed, to create the right consistency for patties.

2. Mold the mixture into 12 small patties and refrigerate them for at least 1 hour to firm up.

3. Pour the sesame seeds onto a plate and gently press the patties into the seeds to coat.

4. In a large skillet over medium-high heat, heat the olive oil.

5. Cook the patties for about 5 minutes, turning once, until they are golden brown on both sides.

Substitution tip: *Chickpeas, green lentils, and white navy beans are all good legumes to make these tasty patties with if red lentils are not available. Use the same amount (2 cups), taking care to mash larger legumes, such as chickpeas, well so the texture stays the same.*

PER SERVING Calories: 374; Total Fat: 23g; Saturated Fat: 4g; Carbohydrates: 29g; Fiber: 11g; Protein: 17g

Sweet Potato Curry

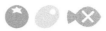

SERVES 4 / PREP TIME: 15 MINUTES / COOK TIME: 25 MINUTES

Curry is an exotic, fragrant meal that can be served over rice or tucked into a pita bread or roti. The sunny color of this curry comes both from the sweet potatoes and the turmeric. Turmeric is a powerful anti-inflammatory that adds a peppery, citrus flavor to the dish.

1 teaspoon extra-virgin olive oil

1 sweet onion, peeled and chopped

2 teaspoons minced garlic

2 teaspoons grated peeled fresh ginger

1 cup sodium-free vegetable stock or broth

3 sweet potatoes, peeled and diced

1 large carrot, peeled and diced

1 tablespoon curry powder

1 teaspoon ground cumin

½ teaspoon ground coriander

½ teaspoon turmeric

1 zucchini, diced

1 yellow squash, diced

1 red bell pepper, thinly sliced

¼ cup water

1 tablespoon cornstarch

1. In a large saucepan over medium-high heat, heat the olive oil.

2. Add the onion, garlic, and ginger and sauté for about 3 minutes until softened.

3. Stir in the vegetable broth, sweet potatoes, carrot, curry powder, cumin, coriander, and turmeric. Bring the liquid to a boil and reduce the heat to low. Simmer for about 15 minutes until the vegetables are tender, stirring occasionally.

4. Add the zucchini, yellow squash, and red bell pepper. Simmer for 5 minutes.

5. In a small bowl, stir together the water and cornstarch until smooth. Stir the cornstarch mixture into the curry, stirring for about 2 minutes until the sauce is thick.

6. Adjust the seasonings as desired and serve.

Ingredient tip: Curry powder is a spice mixture made of many different spices to produce the desired heat and flavor. Try several brands so you get the exact combination that works with a recipe or your own preferences.

PER SERVING Calories: 208; Total Fat: 2g; Saturated Fat: 0g; Carbohydrates: 45g; Fiber: 8g; Protein: 4g

Bell Pepper Frittata with Whole-Wheat Penne

SERVES 4 / PREP TIME: 15 MINUTES / COOK TIME: 30 MINUTES

The addition of whole-wheat penne to a simple frittata creates a meal that is both filling and absolutely delicious. Pasta might not seem like an obvious ingredient in an egg dish, but the slightly chewy texture and nutty flavor works well with the sweet peppers and herbs. You can use any type of pasta you have, such as rotini, macaroni, or farfalle.

5 large eggs

3 large egg whites

½ cup plain Greek yogurt

1 scallion, white and green parts, chopped

1 tablespoon chopped fresh parsley

Pinch sea salt

Pinch freshly ground black pepper

1 tablespoon extra-virgin olive oil

½ cup diced red bell pepper

½ cup diced yellow bell pepper

1 teaspoon minced garlic

2 cups cooked whole-wheat penne

1. Preheat the oven to 350ºF.

2. In a large bowl, whisk the eggs, egg whites, yogurt, scallion, parsley, sea salt, and black pepper. Set aside.

3. In a large ovenproof skillet over medium heat, heat the olive oil.

4. Add the red bell pepper, yellow bell pepper, and garlic. Sauté for about 4 minutes until softened.

5. Add the cooked pasta and stir to mix with the peppers. Use a spatula to arrange the pasta and vegetables evenly in the skillet.

6. Pour the egg mixture into the skillet, shaking gently so the eggs fill in all around the pasta. Cook the eggs for 2 minutes.

7. Transfer the skillet to the oven and bake for about 20 minutes until set and golden brown.

8. Remove from oven and serve.

Variation tip: Warm frittatas are delicious, but this dish can also be fabulous cold tucked in a multigrain wrap or cut into squares for a handy snack. You can even freeze frittata portions and microwave them quickly as a no-hassle breakfast on busy mornings.

PER SERVING Calories: 275; Total Fat: 12g; Saturated Fat: 4g; Carbohydrates: 25g; Fiber: 3g; Protein: 16g

Ratatouille

SERVES 4 / PREP TIME: 15 MINUTES / COOK TIME: 50 MINUTES

Ratatouille, derived from the French word touiller, *"to stir," is a simple dish filled with a mélange of vegetables and fresh herbs. Each vegetable should remain distinct in texture and taste while combining with the others to form a pleasing mixture.*

3 tablespoons extra-virgin olive oil

1 sweet onion, peeled and chopped

1 tablespoon minced garlic

1 large eggplant, cubed

2 zucchini, diced

2 red bell peppers, diced

1 yellow squash, diced

1 (28-ounce) can sodium-free diced tomatoes

2 tablespoons chopped fresh basil

2 tablespoons chopped fresh oregano

Pinch red pepper flakes

Sea salt

Freshly ground black pepper

1. In a large saucepan over medium-high heat, heat the olive oil.

2. Add the onion and garlic, and sauté for about 3 minutes until softened.

3. Add the eggplant and sauté for 15 minutes.

4. Add the zucchini, red bell peppers, yellow squash, tomatoes, basil, oregano, and red pepper flakes to the saucepan and bring the mixture to a boil.

5. Reduce the heat to low, cover, and simmer for about 30 minutes until the vegetables are tender.

6. Season with sea salt and pepper before serving.

Substitution tip: *Four large fresh tomatoes can replace the canned tomatoes. Core and chop the tomatoes into large chunks, and add them along with their juices.*

PER SERVING Calories: 224; Total Fat: 11g; Saturated Fat: 2g; Carbohydrates: 30g; Fiber: 12g; Protein: 6g

Chopped Kale Tabbouleh

SERVES 6 / PREP TIME: 30 MINUTES

Parsley plays a big role in traditional tabbouleh as both a flavor and a vivid splash of color. Parsley is often dismissed as a garnish, but this frilly herb is very nutritious. It's an excellent source of flavonoids, such as luteolin, and vitamin K.

For the dressing

¼ cup extra-virgin olive oil

Juice of 1 lemon

Zest of 1 lemon

Sea salt

Freshly ground black pepper

For the salad

2 cups cooked couscous

2 cups finely chopped kale

1 cup finely chopped cauliflower

1 tomato, seeded and chopped

1 red bell pepper, finely diced

½ English cucumber, finely diced

½ cup red onion, chopped

½ cup chopped fresh parsley

To make the dressing

1. In a small bowl, whisk the olive oil, lemon juice, and lemon zest.

2. Season the dressing with sea salt and pepper. Set aside.

To make the salad

1. In a large bowl, stir together the couscous, kale, cauliflower, tomato, red bell pepper, cucumber, red onion, and parsley.

2. Add the dressing and toss to combine.

3. Serve cold.

Cooking tip: Couscous can be cooked ahead and refrigerated in a covered container for up to 3 days. This is probably the easiest pasta you will ever cook because all you do is add boiling liquid to dried couscous (1:1 ratio), cover, and let sit for about 10 minutes.

PER SERVING Calories: 214; Total Fat: 8g; Saturated Fat: 1g; Carbohydrates: 30g; Fiber: 2g; Protein: 6g

Stuffed Tomatoes

SERVES 4 / PREP TIME: 20 MINUTES , PLUS 30 MINUTES DRAINING /
COOK TIME: 40 MINUTES

The filling for these tomatoes embodies the unique textures and dazzling array of flavors in vegetarian food. Rice, nuts, vegetables, herbs, and a splash of tangy vinegar combine in a balanced and nutritious mixture you might want to eat with a spoon instead of filling the tomatoes. Try roasted unsalted sunflower seeds for an even more complex flavor.

1 teaspoon extra-virgin olive oil, plus more for greasing the baking dish

4 large firm, ripe tomatoes

½ teaspoon sea salt

½ sweet onion, peeled and finely chopped

1 teaspoon minced garlic

1 cup chopped fresh spinach

2 cups cooked brown rice

½ cup sunflower seeds

1 tablespoon balsamic vinegar

2 teaspoons chopped fresh parsley

Sea salt

Freshly ground black pepper

1. Preheat the oven to 350ºF.

2. Lightly grease an 8-by-8-inch baking dish with olive oil and set aside.

3. Carefully cut the tops off the tomatoes, and scoop out the flesh leaving the shell intact. Sprinkle the shells with sea salt, and turn them upside down onto paper towels to drain for 30 minutes.

4. In a large skillet over medium heat, heat the remaining 1 teaspoon of olive oil.

5. Add the onion and garlic, and sauté for about 6 minutes until softened.

6. Add the spinach and sauté for about 2 minutes, or until wilted.

7. Stir in the brown rice, sunflower seeds, balsamic vinegar, and parsley.

8. Season the mixture with sea salt and pepper.

9. Rinse the tomato shells and pat them dry with paper towels.

10. Evenly divide the filling among the tomatoes and place them in the prepared baking dish.

11. Bake for about 30 minutes until the tomatoes are softened and the filling is heated through.

Substitution tip: *Bell peppers in all colors or zucchini make outstanding containers for this filling. If not using tomatoes, skip the salting step and just fill and bake the other vegetables.*

PER SERVING Calories: 264; Total Fat: 6g; Saturated Fat: 1g; Carbohydrates: 47g; Fiber: 5g; Protein: 7g

Pumpkin, Tomato, and Bell Pepper Gratin

SERVES 4 / PREP TIME: 15 MINUTES / COOK TIME: 35 MINUTES

Pumpkin comes in many sizes, ranging from huge ribbon-winning behemoths to small, sweet golden nuggets. Pumpkin is low calorie, contains no saturated fat, is very rich in beta-carotene, iron, potassium, copper, and contains a staggering 246% of the recommended daily allowance of vitamin A in 100 grams (about one-half cup cooked). Pumpkin can help cut the risk of cancer, cardiovascular disease, kidney disease, and promote healthy vision.

2 tablespoons extra-virgin olive oil

1 sweet onion, chopped

2 teaspoons minced garlic

2 cups diced pumpkin or butternut squash

2 red bell peppers, diced

2 tablespoons chopped fresh basil

1 teaspoon chopped fresh oregano

¼ teaspoon sea salt

Pinch ground cloves

4 tomatoes, cut into ¼-inch-thick slices

½ cup crumbled feta cheese

½ cup homemade bread crumbs, or purchased

1. Preheat the oven to 375ºF.

2. In a large skillet over medium-high heat, heat the olive oil.

3. Add the onion and garlic, and sauté for about 3 minutes until softened.

4. Add the pumpkin and red bell peppers. Sauté for about 10 minutes more until the vegetables are tender.

5. Remove from the heat and stir in the basil, oregano, sea salt, and cloves. Spoon the pumpkin mixture into a 9-by-13-inch baking dish.

6. Layer the tomato slices on top.

7. In a small bowl, stir together the feta cheese and bread crumbs until crumbly. Top the casserole with the feta mixture and bake for about 20 minutes until golden and crisp.

Ingredient tip: *Sometimes the only pumpkins you can find are large ones that leave lots of leftover flesh. Cut the leftover pumpkin into chunks and place them on baking trays in the freezer until frozen. Transfer the frozen chunks to freezer-safe bags and keep frozen for up to 3 months.*

PER SERVING Calories: 209; Total Fat: 11g; Saturated Fat: 3g; Carbohydrates: 26g; Fiber: 5g; Protein: 6g

Wheat Berry–Stuffed Acorn Squash

SERVES 4 / PREP TIME: 15 MINUTES / COOK TIME: 55 MINUTES

Wheat berries consist of the entire wheat kernel, including the germ, bran, and endosperm. Wheat berries are chewy when cooked and make a brilliant alternative to rice, legumes, and pasta. This grain is prepared in boiling water or stock, and can keep refrigerated for up to 4 days in a sealed container.

2 acorn squash, halved and seeded

2 tablespoons extra-virgin olive oil, plus more for greasing squash

1 sweet onion, chopped

1 teaspoon minced garlic

2 cups cooked wheat berries

½ cup shredded carrot

½ cup chopped almonds

½ cup dried cranberries

2 teaspoons freshly squeezed lemon juice

1 teaspoon ground cumin

½ teaspoon ground coriander

2 teaspoons chopped fresh cilantro

1. Preheat the oven to 400°F.

2. Line a baking sheet with aluminum foil.

3. Lightly brush the cut side of the squash with oil and place them cut-side down on the prepared sheet. Roast the squash for about 45 minutes until tender.

4. While the squash is roasting, in a large skillet over medium heat, heat the 2 tablespoons of olive oil.

5. Add the onion and garlic, and sauté for about 3 minutes until softened.

6. Stir in the wheat berries, carrot, almonds, cranberries, lemon juice, cumin, and coriander.

7. Remove the squash from the oven. Spoon the wheat berry filling into the squash, return to the oven, and bake for 5 minutes.

8. Garnish with cilantro and serve.

Cooking tip: *Acorn squash is very hard and can be dangerous to cut because it often rolls when pressed with a knife. Microwave the squash for 1 to 2 minutes on high to create a softer, easier-to-cut vegetable.*

PER SERVING Calories: 292; Total Fat: 14g; Saturated Fat: 2g; Carbohydrates: 41g; Fiber: 6g; Protein: 7g

Broiled Portobello Mushroom Burgers with Goat Cheese

  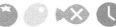

SERVES 4 / PREP TIME: 15 MINUTES / COOK TIME: 5 MINUTES

Portobello mushrooms seem designed to fit perfectly on hamburger buns as a burger substitute. These mushrooms are large, with a meaty texture that holds up beautifully under a broiler or on a grill. Portobellos are low in fat and calories, and high in protein, fiber, potassium, and vitamin D.

4 large portobello mushroom caps

1 red onion, cut into ¼-inch-thick slices

2 tablespoons extra-virgin olive oil

2 tablespoons balsamic vinegar

Pinch sea salt

¼ cup goat cheese

¼ cup chopped sun-dried tomatoes

4 ciabatta buns

1 cup shredded kale

1. Preheat the oven to broil.

2. In a large bowl, toss the mushroom caps and onion slices with the olive oil, balsamic vinegar, and sea salt. Place the caps, bottom-side up, and the onion slices on a baking sheet.

3. Broil for about 5 minutes until the vegetables are tender and lightly caramelized. Remove the vegetables from the oven, transfer to a plate, and set aside.

4. In a small bowl, stir together the goat cheese and sun-dried tomatoes until well blended.

5. Toast the buns under the broiler for about 30 seconds until golden.

6. Spread the goat cheese mixture on each bun top.

7. Place a mushroom cap and onion slice on each bun bottom and cover with shredded kale.

8. Put the buns together and serve.

Cooking tip: *Kale needs to sit for at least 5 to 10 minutes after you cut or tear it because the leaves produce an antioxidant to repair the damage. This antioxidant makes the kale healthier for you.*

PER SERVING Calories: 327; Total Fat: 11g; Saturated Fat: 3g; Carbohydrates: 49g; Fiber: 4g; Protein: 11g

Classic Colcannon

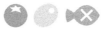

SERVES 4 / PREP TIME: 10 MINUTES / COOK TIME: 50 MINUTES

Colcannon is a traditional Irish dish made with potatoes and shredded cabbage or kale. The inexpensive ingredients combine beautifully to create a rib-sticking casserole that tastes even better the next day. If you don't need a vegetarian dish, top the casserole with lean sausages before baking it in the oven.

4 russet potatoes, peeled and cut into 1-inch chunks

2 tablespoons extra-virgin olive oil

½ sweet onion, thinly sliced

1 teaspoon minced garlic

6 cups finely shredded cabbage

¼ cup chopped fresh parsley

Pinch sea salt

1. Place the potatoes in a large saucepan and cover them with cold water by about 1½ inches. Bring to a boil over high heat. Reduce the heat to low and simmer the potatoes for about 30 minutes until tender. Drain and mash until fluffy.

2. While the potatoes cook, heat the olive oil in a large skillet over medium-high heat.

3. Add the onion and garlic, and sauté for about 3 minutes until softened.

4. Add the cabbage to the skillet and sauté for about 15 minutes more until the cabbage is tender.

5. Stir the cabbage mixture and the parsley into the mashed potatoes.

6. Season with the sea salt and serve.

Substitution tip: *Sweet potatoes, celeriac, yams, or a combination can be used instead of potatoes for a unique variation on this classic dish. Use the same amount of starchy vegetables so the texture is perfect.*

PER SERVING Calories: 241; Total Fat: 7g; Saturated Fat: 1g; Carbohydrates: 41g; Fiber: 8g; Protein: 5g

Green Bean Stew (Lubya bi-Zayt)

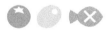

SERVES 4 / PREP TIME: 10 MINUTES / COOK TIME: 40 MINUTES

This dish, known as "Lubya bi-Zayt" in Arabic, or green beans in olive oil, is a traditional vegetarian Lebanese recipe. The green beans should be nice and soft when finished.

¼ cup extra-virgin olive oil

3 garlic cloves, chopped

1 sweet onion, chopped

Sea salt

Freshly ground black pepper

1 pound fresh green beans, ends snipped and cut into 2-inch pieces

1 (8-ounce) can tomato sauce

½ cup water

1. In a small skillet over medium heat, heat the olive oil.
2. Add the garlic and onion, and sauté for about 3 minutes until the garlic is fragrant and the onion softens.
3. Season with sea salt and pepper.
4. Add the beans to the skillet, stirring gently with a wooden spoon. Cover and cook for 10 minutes.
5. Stir in the tomato sauce and water. Cover again and cook for 25 minutes.

Serving tip: Serve this as a side dish or over rice. It can also be enjoyed with pita bread.

PER SERVING Calories: 159; Total Fat: 13g; Saturated Fat: 2g; Carbohydrates: 12g; Fiber: 5g; Protein: 3g

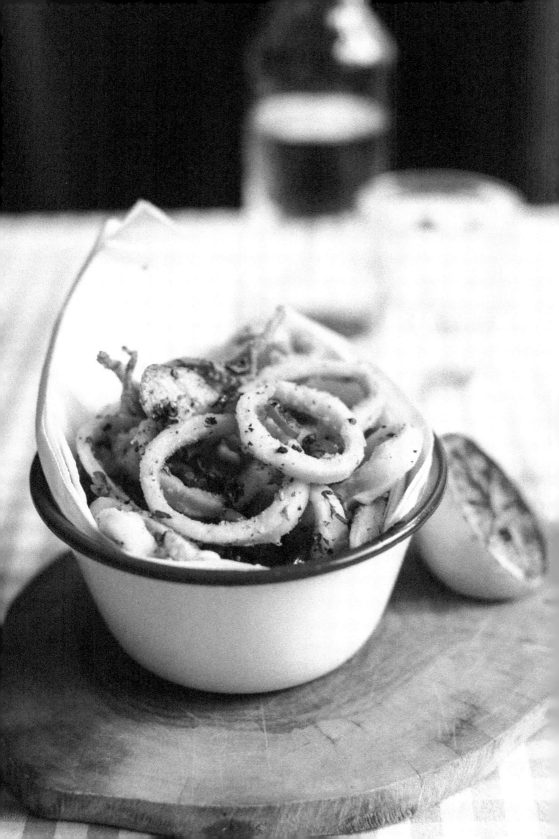

CHAPTER 9

Seafood

Broiled Chili Calamari

SERVES 4 / PREP TIME: 10 MINUTES, PLUS 1 HOUR MARINATING / COOK TIME: 8 MINUTES

Calamari is an appetizer made from squid, a marine cephalopod. Squid—nutritional bonanza for those looking to eat healthy—is a superb source of protein, copper, selenium, phosphorus, vitamin B_{12}, and zinc. Try barbecuing the squid sections instead of broiling, for an incomparable smoky flavor.

2 tablespoons extra-virgin olive oil

1 teaspoon chili powder

½ teaspoon ground cumin

Zest of 1 lime

Juice of 1 lime

Dash sea salt

Dash freshly ground black pepper

1½ pounds squid, cleaned and split open, with tentacles cut into ½-inch rounds

2 tablespoons chopped cilantro

2 tablespoons minced red bell pepper

1. In a medium bowl, stir together the olive oil, chili powder, cumin, lime zest, lime juice, sea salt, and pepper.
2. Add the squid to the marinade and stir to coat. Cover and refrigerate for 1 hour.
3. Preheat the oven to broil.
4. Arrange the squid on a baking sheet. Broil for about 8 minutes, turning once, until tender.
5. Garnish the broiled calamari with cilantro and red bell pepper and serve.

Substitution tip: If you don't want to clean the squid yourself, ask the fish counter staff to do it or buy the squid precut, fresh or frozen.

PER SERVING Calories: 222; Total Fat: 10g; Saturated Fat: 2g; Carbohydrates: 6g; Fiber: 0g; Protein: 27g

Mussels in Spicy Tomato Sauce

SERVES 4 / PREP TIME: 20 MINUTES / COOK TIME: 15 MINUTES

Mussels have been eaten for more than 20,000 years around the world and cultivated in beds for almost 1,000 years. They are an outstanding source of protein, omega-3 fatty acids, and iron. Fifteen mussels have as much protein as a 6-ounce steak!

2 tablespoons extra-virgin olive oil

½ sweet onion, finely chopped

1 jalapeño pepper, seeded and finely chopped

2 teaspoons minced garlic

2 tomatoes, finely chopped

½ cup white wine

Zest of 1 lemon

Juice of 1 lemon

3 pounds mussels, scrubbed and debearded

¼ cup chopped fresh parsley

1. In a large, deep skillet over medium heat, heat the olive oil.

2. Add the onion, jalapeño, and garlic, and sauté for about 3 minutes until softened.

3. Stir in the tomatoes, white wine, lemon zest, and lemon juice. Bring to a boil and then reduce the heat to low. Simmer for about 5 minutes until the sauce is thick.

4. Add the mussels to the sauce. Cover and simmer for about 5 minutes, shaking the pan occasionally, until the shells open.

5. Discard any unopened shells and serve the mussels with the sauce, topped with parsley.

Cooking tip: To debeard mussels, pull off the long hairy pieces called byssal threads toward the hinge end of the mussel rather than the front, or you will kill the mussel and it will become inedible.

PER SERVING Calories: 398; Total Fat: 15g; Saturated Fat: 3g; Carbohydrates: 18g; Fiber: 1g; Protein: 41g

Scallops in Three-Citrus Sauce

SERVES 4 / PREP TIME: 10 MINUTES / COOK TIME: 15 MINUTES

Scallops are available year-round and come in several sizes—from small bay scallops to the larger sea scallops. Scallops are a first-rate source of vitamin B$_{12}$, protein, selenium, and magnesium.

2 teaspoons extra-virgin olive oil

1 shallot, minced

20 sea scallops, cleaned

1 tablespoon lemon zest

2 teaspoons orange zest

1 teaspoon lime zest

1 tablespoon chopped fresh basil

½ cup freshly squeezed orange juice

2 tablespoons freshly squeezed lemon juice

2 tablespoons honey

1 tablespoon plain Greek yogurt

Pinch sea salt

1. In a large skillet over medium-high heat, heat the olive oil.

2. Add the shallot and sauté for about 1 minute until softened.

3. Place the scallops in the skillet and pan sear for about 5 minutes, turning once, until tender.

4. Move the scallops to the edge of the skillet and stir in the lemon, orange, and lime zests; basil; orange juice; and lemon juice.

5. Simmer the sauce for about 3 minutes and then whisk in the honey, yogurt, and sea salt.

6. Cook the sauce for 4 minutes more and then coat the scallops in the sauce and serve.

Ingredient tip: Scallops need to be carefully prepared to ensure the best results. Always remove the side muscle because it is tough and rub the entire surface of the scallop to remove any accumulated grit. Running each scallop under cold water is the best way to clean them thoroughly.

PER SERVING Calories: 207; Total Fat: 4g; Saturated Fat: 1g; Carbohydrates: 17g; Fiber: 0g; Protein: 26g

Shrimp and Vegetable Packets

SERVES 4 / PREP TIME: 15 MINUTES / COOK TIME: 20 MINUTES

Shrimp is an extremely popular seafood because it is sweet and succulent, as well as easy to prepare using many different cooking methods, such as grilling, braising, poaching, and sautéing. Shrimp is low in fat and calories, and high in protein, phosphorus, selenium, and B_{12}. Eating shrimp regularly can reduce the risk of many diseases, including type 2 diabetes, cancer, and heart disease.

½ pound baby potatoes, quartered

2 large carrots, peeled and cut into batons (thin sticks)

1 red bell pepper, cut into strips

8 baby bok choy, washed thoroughly and quartered

4 shallots, peeled and quartered

2 pounds (16 to 20 count) shrimp, peeled and deveined

2 tablespoons extra-virgin olive oil

1 tablespoon chopped fresh parsley

1 tablespoon chopped fresh thyme

Sea salt

Freshly ground black pepper

1. Preheat the oven to 425ºF.

2. Cut 4 sheets of aluminum foil, each about 12 inches long, and lay them on the counter.

3. Divide the potatoes, carrots, red bell pepper, bok choy, and shallots among the 4 foil sheets.

4. Top the vegetables with the shrimp, dividing it evenly.

5. Drizzle the packets with olive oil and sprinkle each with parsley, thyme, sea salt, and pepper.

6. Fold the foil over the shrimp and vegetables, covering all the ingredients completely, and seal the packets closed.

7. Place the packets on a baking sheet and place them in the oven. Bake for about 20 minutes until the shrimp is cooked through and the vegetables are tender.

Ingredient tip: Shrimp currently has a bad reputation because much of it is not sustainably caught and farm-raised crustaceans are produced under questionable farming techniques. Look for shrimp labeled by the Marine Stewardship Council or other accredited agencies to ensure a sustainable product.

PER SERVING Calories: 414; Total Fat: 11g; Saturated Fat: 2g; Carbohydrates: 25g; Fiber: 5g; Protein: 56g

Broiled Salmon with Avocado Pico de Gallo

SERVES 4 / PREP TIME: 15 MINUTES / COOK TIME: 15 MINUTES

Salmon is the poster fish for healthy diets because it is incredibly rich in omega-3 fatty acids, selenium, calcium, and vitamin A. Salmon can help decrease inflammation, boost your metabolism, reduce the risk of Alzheimer's, and promote a healthy cardiovascular system. Salmon also promotes skin and hair health.

For the pico de gallo

1 tomato, diced

1 avocado, peeled, pitted, and diced

1 jalapeño pepper, seeded and minced

½ cup corn kernels

2 tablespoons chopped red onion

1 tablespoon chopped fresh cilantro

1 tablespoon freshly squeezed lime juice

Pinch sea salt

For the fish

½ teaspoon ground coriander

½ teaspoon ground cumin

¼ teaspoon paprika

Pinch sea salt

Pinch freshly ground black pepper

4 (5-ounce) boneless skinless salmon fillets

To make the pico de gallo

In a medium bowl, stir together the tomato, avocado, jalapeño, corn, red onion, cilantro, lime juice, and sea salt. Set aside.

To make the fish

1. Preheat the oven to broil.

2. In a small bowl, stir together the coriander, cumin, paprika, sea salt, and pepper until well mixed.

3. Rub the salmon with the spice mix and place the fillets on a baking sheet.

4. Broil, turning once, for about 15 minutes until just cooked through.

5. Serve the salmon topped with the avocado pico de gallo.

Ingredient tip: *Don't ignore those hard, unripened avocados. This fruit does not ripen until after it is picked. You can ripen an avocado quickly by exposing it to the naturally occurring gas called ethylene, produced by bananas and apples. Just pop the avocado in a paper bag with these other fruits and it will ripen quickly.*

PER SERVING Calories: 313; Total Fat: 18g; Saturated Fat: 3g; Carbohydrates: 10g; Fiber: 4g; Protein: 29g

Citrus-Poached Salmon

SERVES 4 / PREP TIME: 10 MINUTES / COOK TIME: 40 MINUTES

Herbs are commonly used for cooking applications, so it is easy to forget they were, for centuries, used as medicine. Thyme adds a light, almost licorice, flavor to the poaching liquid and is a fabulous source of copper, iron, and vitamins A and C. Thyme was prescribed for congestion and cough, so perhaps this salmon dish would be appropriate during cold season.

6 cups water

½ cup freshly squeezed lemon juice

Juice of 1 lime

Zest of 1 lime

1 sweet onion, thinly sliced

1 cup coarsely chopped celery leaves

1 tablespoon chopped fresh dill

1 tablespoon chopped fresh thyme

2 dried bay leaves

½ teaspoon black peppercorns

½ teaspoon sea salt

1 (24-ounce) salmon side, skinned, deboned, and cut into 4 pieces

1. In a large saucepan over medium-high heat, stir together the water, lemon juice, lime juice, lime zest, onion, celery greens, dill, thyme, bay leaves, peppercorns, and sea salt. Bring to a boil and then reduce the heat to low. Simmer the poaching liquid for 30 minutes.

2. Strain the liquid through a fine-mesh sieve, discarding the solids.

3. Pour the strained poaching liquid into a large skillet over low heat and bring to a simmer.

4. Add the fish, cover the skillet, and poach the fish for about 10 minutes until it is opaque and just cooked through. Carefully remove the salmon from the liquid.

5. Serve warm or cold.

Ingredient tip: *Farmed salmon is common because it is inexpensive and available year-round. Wild-caught salmon is worth the price, though it costs more because it is higher in omega-3 fatty acids, minerals, and vitamins.*

PER SERVING Calories: 248; Total Fat: 11g; Saturated Fat: 2g; Carbohydrates: 4g; Fiber: 1g; Protein: 34g

Trout with Wilted Greens

SERVES 4 / PREP TIME: 5 MINUTES / COOK TIME: 15 MINUTES

This dish is so simple to prepare yet full of complex flavors. A generous squeeze of lemon juice brightens the flavor of the kale and accents the trout. Kale does not overpower the taste of the trout. Spinach, beet greens, and arugula can all be used instead of or with the kale.

2 teaspoons extra-virgin olive oil, plus more for greasing the dish

2 cups chopped kale

2 cups chopped Swiss chard

½ sweet onion, thinly sliced

4 (5-ounce) boneless skin-on trout fillets

Juice of 1 lemon

Sea salt

Freshly ground black pepper

Zest of 1 lemon

1. Preheat the oven to 375°F.
2. Lightly grease a 9-by-13-inch baking dish with olive oil.
3. Arrange the kale, Swiss chard, and onion in the dish.
4. Top the greens with the fish, skin-side up, and drizzle the fish with olive oil and lemon juice.
5. Season the fish with sea salt and pepper, and bake for about 15 minutes until the fish flakes easily with a fork.
6. Sprinkle with lemon zest and serve.

Ingredient tip: Most supermarket fish counters have large tanks filled with rainbow trout, so adventurous patrons can select very fresh fish. The fishmonger will clean, gut, and skin it for you while you finish your shopping.

PER SERVING Calories: 315; Total Fat: 14g; Saturated Fat: 2g; Carbohydrates: 6g; Fiber: 1g; Protein: 39g

Pistachio-Crusted Sole

SERVES 4 / PREP TIME: 10 MINUTES / COOK TIME: 10 MINUTES

Nut crusts pair beautifully with fish because lean fish benefits from the fat in the nuts. Since fish cooks so quickly, nuts don't have time to burn, either. This is a very quick meal that can be made even more quickly when you put the entire recipe together in the morning, store it in the refrigerator, and pop it in the oven when you get home from work.

4 (5-ounce) boneless sole fillets
Sea salt
Freshly ground black pepper
½ cup finely chopped pistachios

Zest of 1 lemon
Juice of 1 lemon
1 teaspoon extra-virgin olive oil

1. Preheat the oven to 350°F.
2. Line a baking sheet with parchment paper and set aside.
3. Pat the fish dry with paper towels and lightly season with sea salt and pepper.
4. In a small bowl, stir together the pistachios and lemon zest.
5. Place the sole on the prepared sheet and press about 2 tablespoons of the pistachio mixture on top of each fillet.
6. Drizzle the fish with lemon juice and olive oil.
7. Bake for about 10 minutes until the topping is golden and the fish flakes easily with a fork.

Substitution tip: Use chopped almond, hazelnuts, pecans, or cashews instead of pistachios. Sesame seeds, sunflower seeds, and pumpkin seeds also make a great coating for sole.

PER SERVING Calories: 166; Total Fat: 6g; Saturated Fat: 1g; Carbohydrates: 2g; Fiber: 1g; Protein: 26g

Stuffed Sole Fillets

SERVES 4 / PREP TIME: 20 MINUTES / COOK TIME: 25 MINUTES

Crab is the main ingredient of this rich filling and is considered a healthy eating choice despite the fact that it is naturally high in sodium. Even if you avoid sodium, you can still enjoy this dish because each portion uses only 2 tablespoons of crab. Crab is low in fat and calories, and an excellent source of vitamin B_{12} and protein.

1 tablespoon extra-virgin olive oil, plus more for greasing the dish

½ pound crabmeat, flaked

¼ pound chopped cooked shrimp

¼ cup homemade bread crumbs

¼ cup plain Greek yogurt

1 scallion, white and green parts, chopped

1 tablespoon freshly squeezed lemon juice

Pinch sea salt

Pinch freshly ground black pepper

4 sole fillets

1. Preheat the oven to 375°F.
2. Lightly grease a 9-by-13-inch baking dish with olive oil.
3. In a medium bowl, stir together the crabmeat, shrimp, bread crumbs, yogurt, scallion, lemon juice, sea salt, and pepper until well mixed.

4. Lay the fillets flat on a work surface. Evenly divide the filling among the fish. Roll up the fillets and place them seam-side down in the baking dish.

5. Drizzle the olive oil over the fish and bake for about 25 minutes until the fish flakes easily with a fork.

Ingredient tip: Getting crabmeat out of the legs and claws can be hard and buying fresh crab can be expensive. Look for good-quality canned crab that has no added salt and is labeled blue or Dungeness crab.

PER SERVING Calories: 275; Total Fat: 8g; Saturated Fat: 2g; Carbohydrates: 15g; Fiber: 1g; Protein: 37g

Pan-Seared Haddock with Olive-Tomato Sauce

SERVES 4 / PREP TIME: 10 MINUTES / COOK TIME: 20 MINUTES

Haddock is a popular saltwater fish with a silky texture and firm white flesh. It is a common choice for fish and chips in the UK and North America. Avoid haddock that is opaque and has loose flesh, because it is not fresh. Haddock is high in protein, potassium, phosphorus, and vitamin B_3.

4 (6-ounce) boneless skinless haddock fillets

Pinch sea salt

Pinch freshly ground black pepper

2 tablespoons extra-virgin olive oil

2 shallots, chopped

1 teaspoon minced garlic

1 (15-ounce) can sodium-free diced tomatoes

¼ cup sliced Kalamata olives

2 tablespoons chopped fresh parsley

1. Season the fish with sea salt and pepper.

2. In a large skillet over medium-high heat, heat 1 tablespoon of the olive oil.

3. Add the fish and panfry for about 5 minutes per side, or until it flakes easily with a fork. Transfer to a plate, cover it to keep warm, and set aside.

4. Wipe the skillet with a paper towel and place it back over medium-high heat. Add the remaining 1 tablespoon of olive oil, the shallots, and garlic. Sauté for about 3 minutes until softened.

5. Stir in the tomatoes, olives, and parsley. Cook the sauce for 5 minutes, or until heated through.

6. Serve the fish topped with the tomato sauce.

Substitution tip: *Any firm-fleshed white fish will work with this tangy tomato sauce. Halibut, sea bass, cod, or tilapia all have enough texture and flavor.*

PER SERVING Calories: 288; Total Fat: 10g; Saturated Fat: 2g; Carbohydrates: 6g; Fiber: 2g; Protein: 43g

Tilapia with Fresh Veggie Salsa

SERVES 4 / PREP TIME: 15 MINUTES / COOK TIME: 10 MINUTES

Tilapia is the fish of choice for many home cooks because it is inexpensive and available year-round. Most tilapia found in the supermarket, unless otherwise labeled, is farmed, which can mean it contains antibiotics or other contaminants. Try to source wild caught whenever possible or limit tilapia to one meal per week.

For the veggie salsa

½ cup diced English cucumber

½ cup diced yellow squash

½ cup diced orange bell pepper

8 cherry tomatoes, quartered

1 scallion, white and green parts, finely chopped

1 teaspoon chopped fresh cilantro

Zest of 1 lime

Juice of 1 lime

Sea salt

Freshly ground black pepper

For the fish

¼ cup whole-wheat flour

4 (6-ounce) tilapia fillets

2 teaspoons extra-virgin olive oil

To make the veggie salsa

1. In a medium bowl, stir together the cucumber, yellow squash, orange bell pepper, tomatoes, scallion, cilantro, lime zest, and lime juice.

2. Season with sea salt and pepper. Set aside.

To make the fish

1. Place the flour on a plate.
2. Pat the fish dry with paper towels and then dredge it in the flour, coating both sides.
3. In a large skillet over medium-high heat, heat the olive oil.
4. Add the tilapia and panfry for about 5 minutes per side until golden brown.
5. Serve immediately topped with one or two heaping spoonfuls of salsa.

Ingredient tip: *If you have only regular cucumbers instead of English, peel them before using in the salsa because the skin is often coated with wax, bitter, and unpalatably thick.*

PER SERVING Calories: 242; Total Fat: 5g; Saturated Fat: 1g; Carbohydrates: 17g; Fiber: 4g; Protein: 35g

Hearty Fish Chowder

SERVES 8 / PREP TIME: 15 MINUTES / COOK TIME: 25 MINUTES

As with any multi-ingredient soup or stew, tailor the fish and vegetables to suit your refrigerator contents and taste. Salmon, scallops, shrimp, other types of fish, and mussels can be added for a truly eclectic chowder. Just check to see how long each protein needs to cook so you don't overcook or undercook any additions.

1 tablespoon extra-virgin olive oil

1½ sweet onions, peeled and chopped

3 large celery stalks with leaves, diced

8 cups sodium-free vegetable or fish stock, or broth

1 (28-ounce) can sodium-free diced tomatoes, with juice

2 carrots, peeled and cut into disks

2 large sweet potatoes, peeled and diced

24 ounces firm white-fleshed fish, cubed

2 cups green beans, cut into 1-inch pieces

Pinch red pepper flakes

Sea salt

Freshly ground black pepper

¼ cup water

2 tablespoons cornstarch

2 tablespoons chopped fresh parsley

1. In a large saucepan over medium-high heat, heat the olive oil.

2. Add the onions and celery, and sauté for about 4 minutes until softened.

3. Stir in the stock, tomatoes, carrots, and sweet potatoes. Bring to a boil and then reduce the heat to low. Simmer for about 10 minutes until the vegetables are crisp-tender.

4. Add the fish, green beans, and red pepper flakes. Simmer for about 5 minutes more until the fish is just cooked through.

5. Season the chowder with sea salt and pepper.

6. In a small bowl, whisk together the water and cornstarch. Stir this into the hot soup, stirring gently for about 3 minutes until the chowder thickens.

7. Garnish with the parsley and serve.

Cooking tip: If you want to freeze the chowder, leave out the green beans because they will get too soft when you reheat the soup.

PER SERVING Calories: 280; Total Fat: 5g; Saturated Fat: 1g; Carbohydrates: 24g; Fiber: 4g; Protein: 24g

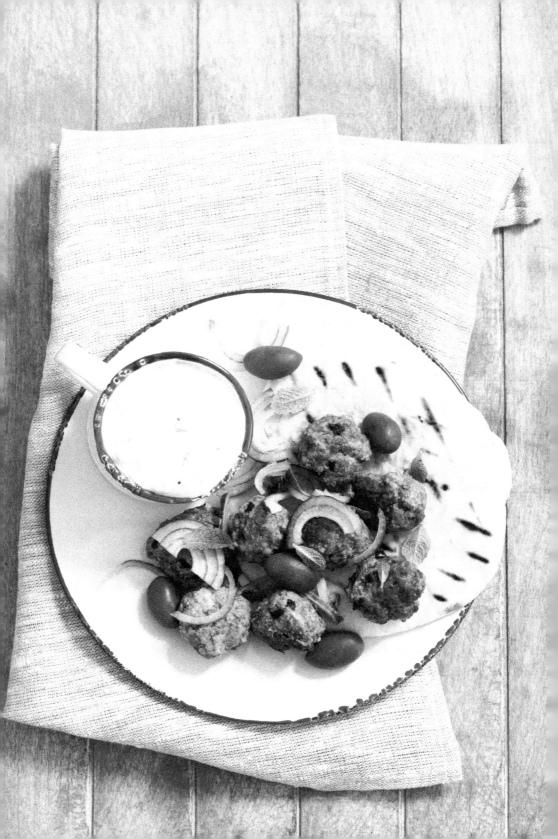

CHAPTER 10

Poultry

Chicken Cassoulet

SERVES 6 / PREP TIME: 10 MINUTES / COOK TIME: 20 MINUTES

Cassoulet is a white bean stew cooked in an earthenware pot called a cassole. Don't worry if you don't have one because you can still make a tempting cassoulet on your stove top. If you want a more authentic feel, bake this stew in the oven in a covered skillet.

2 teaspoons extra-virgin olive oil

½ sweet onion, chopped

2 teaspoons minced garlic

1 cup sodium-free chicken stock or broth

2 cups diced cooked chicken breast

2 cups cooked Great Northern beans

2 cups cooked black beans

1 cup cooked lentils

2 teaspoons chopped fresh oregano

1 teaspoon smoked paprika

1 teaspoon ground cumin

¼ teaspoon cayenne pepper

4 cups chopped kale, thoroughly washed

Sea salt

Freshly ground black pepper

1. In a large saucepan over medium-high heat, heat the olive oil.

2. Add the onion and garlic, and sauté for about 2 minutes until softened.

3. Stir in the chicken stock, cooked chicken, Northern beans, black beans, lentils, oregano, smoked paprika, cumin, and cayenne pepper. Bring to a boil and then reduce the heat to low. Simmer for 15 minutes.

4. Stir in the kale and simmer for about 3 minutes until the greens are wilted.

5. Season with sea salt and pepper and serve.

Substitution tip: Omit the chicken breast and use vegetable stock to create a delicious vegetarian and vegan dish.

PER SERVING Calories: 285; Total Fat: 5g; Saturated Fat: 0g; Carbohydrates: 34g; Fiber: 8g; Protein: 28g

Chicken Florentine Casserole

SERVES 6 / PREP TIME: 10 MINUTES / COOK TIME: 30 MINUTES

Casseroles are cooking magic: you place all your ingredients in one big dish, bake them, and out pops a mouthwatering meal. You can even make the whole thing ahead of time and have absolutely no cleanup the day you serve it. Casseroles are very forgiving, so if you are missing an ingredient, such as the mushrooms or zucchini, simply add something else.

1 tablespoon extra-virgin olive oil, plus more for greasing the dish

1 sweet onion, peeled and chopped

1 cup sliced button mushrooms

1 cup diced zucchini

2 teaspoons minced garlic

1 tablespoon all-purpose flour

1 cup milk

½ cup grated Asiago cheese

⅛ teaspoon ground nutmeg

⅛ teaspoon freshly ground black pepper

2 (6-ounce) cooked boneless skinless chicken breasts, chopped

2 cups cooked brown rice

2 cups packed fresh spinach

1. Preheat the oven to 350ºF.

2. Lightly grease a 9-by-13-inch baking dish with olive oil and set aside.

3. In a medium saucepan over medium-high heat, heat the 1 tablespoon of olive oil.

4. Add the onion, mushrooms, zucchini, and garlic. Sauté for about 5 minutes until softened.

5. Stir in the flour and then stir in the milk, whisking for about 5 minutes until the sauce thickens.

6. Whisk in the Asiago cheese, nutmeg, and pepper. Transfer the sauce to a large bowl.

7. Stir in the chicken, brown rice, and spinach until well mixed.

8. Spoon the chicken mixture into the prepared dish. Bake for about 20 minutes until lightly browned and bubbly.

Ingredient tip: *Stay away from larger zucchini because they are fibrous and have many bitter seeds. Look for vegetables with unblemished, shiny skin that feel heavier than their size.*

PER SERVING Calories: 272; Total Fat: 8g; Saturated Fat: 1g; Carbohydrates: 36g; Fiber: 2g; Protein: 20g

Golden Chicken with Cucumber-Yogurt Sauce

SERVES 4 / PREP TIME: 10 MINUTES / COOK TIME: 20 MINUTES

The creamy, fresh sauce coating the chicken in this dish is basically tzatziki sauce with a twist. If you end up with extra—which is not likely because it is tasty enough to eat with a spoon—use the sauce as a dip or sandwich dressing. If you double or triple the recipe, this citrus-spiked delight could be a refreshing side salad for grilled pork or salmon.

For the sauce

1 cup shredded cucumber, with the liquid squeezed out

½ cup plain Greek yogurt

Zest of 1 lemon

Juice of 1 lemon

1 tablespoon honey

2 teaspoons chopped fresh chives

Pinch sea salt

Pinch freshly ground black pepper

For the chicken

1 tablespoon extra-virgin olive oil

4 (5-ounce) boneless skinless chicken breasts

Dash hot paprika

Sea salt

Freshly ground black pepper

To make the sauce

In a small bowl, stir together the cucumber, yogurt, lemon zest, lemon juice, honey, chives, sea salt, and pepper. Set aside.

To make the chicken

1. Preheat the oven to 400ºF.

2. In a medium ovenproof skillet over medium-high heat, heat the olive oil.

3. Season the chicken breasts with hot paprika, sea salt, and pepper.

4. Add the chicken to the skillet and pan sear for about 3 minutes per side until lightly browned.

5. Place the skillet in the oven and roast the chicken for about 15 minutes, or until cooked through.

6. Serve with a generous scoop of Cucumber-Yogurt Sauce.

Ingredient tip: *Experiment with the honey you use in your recipes because the types of flowers that the bees collect nectar from affect the flavor and color of the honey. Buckwheat honey is darker and stronger, while alfalfa honey is very floral and pale.*

PER SERVING Calories: 262; Total Fat: 10g; Saturated Fat: 4g; Carbohydrates: 9g; Fiber: 0g; Protein: 33g

Pecan-Crusted Chicken

SERVES 4 / PREP TIME: 20 MINUTES / COOK TIME: 25 TO 30 MINUTES

Pecans make an attractive breading for mild-tasting chicken breast and this coating locks in the juiciness. Pecans are not true nuts; rather, botanically they are fruit, very high in phyto-nutrients, vitamins, and minerals. Pecans have been linked to lower LDL cholesterol and increased HDL cholesterol, as well as protecting the body from disease.

4 (4-ounce) boneless skinless chicken breasts

Sea salt

½ cup all-purpose flour

2 large eggs

½ cup ground pecans

2 tablespoons extra-virgin olive oil

1. Preheat the oven to 350°F.
2. Line a baking sheet with parchment paper and set aside.
3. Pat the chicken dry on both sides and lightly season with sea salt.
4. Place the flour on a plate.
5. In a small bowl, whisk the eggs and place it beside the flour.

6. Place the ground pecans on another plate and set it next to the beaten eggs.

7. Dredge 1 chicken breast first in the flour, next dip it into the eggs, and then dredge it in the pecans until coated. Place the coated breast on the prepared sheet.

8. Repeat the three steps with the remaining chicken breasts.

9. Brush the chicken lightly with olive oil and bake for 25 to 30 minutes, or until the chicken is golden brown and cooked through, turning once.

Cooking tip: *Cut the chicken breasts into strips and make kid-friendly chicken fingers instead of coating full breasts. The cooking time will be about 5 minutes less for the fingers.*

PER SERVING Calories: 435; Total Fat: 25g; Saturated Fat: 5g; Carbohydrates: 13g; Fiber: 1g; Protein: 38g

Chicken Piccata

SERVES 4 / PREP TIME: 10 MINUTES / COOK TIME: 30 MINUTES

Piccata *refers to a method of preparing meat or chicken that slices the protein thinly, coating it, sautéing it, and, finally, serving the golden brown meat or poultry with a sauce. Capers and lemon are common accents for the simple sauce. This dish would also be lovely made with veal or pork.*

¼ cup whole-wheat flour

½ teaspoon freshly ground black pepper

¼ teaspoon sea salt

4 (4-ounce) boneless skinless chicken breasts, halved widthwise

2 tablespoons extra-virgin olive oil

¾ cup sodium-free chicken stock or broth

Zest of 1 lemon

Juice of 1 lemon

1 tablespoon capers

1. In a small bowl, stir together the flour, pepper, and sea salt.

2. Dredge the chicken in the flour and set aside on a plate.

3. In a large skillet over medium-high heat, heat the olive oil.

4. Add the chicken and cook for about 8 minutes, turning once, until the chicken is browned on both sides. Transfer to a plate and set aside.

5. Add the chicken stock, lemon zest, lemon juice, and capers to the skillet and bring the liquid to a boil. Reduce the heat to low and simmer for about 10 minutes, or until the sauce reduces by one-third.

6. Return the chicken to the skillet, turning to coat it in the sauce, and simmer for about 10 minutes more until the chicken is cooked through and tender.

Ingredient tip: Capers are the flower buds of a plant native to the Mediterranean region. For this dish, try to find the smaller size, called nonpareil, because they are milder in flavor.

PER SERVING Calories: 283; Total Fat: 11g; Saturated Fat: 1g; Carbohydrates: 6g; Fiber: 0g; Protein: 38g

Tuscan Chicken and Rice

SERVES 6 / PREP TIME: 20 MINUTES / COOK TIME: 45 MINUTES

Italian food traditions vary depending on the region, and Tuscan is characterized by olive oil, fresh herbs, simply prepared vegetables, and less use of pasta. The rice in this dish is not strictly Tuscan, but it soaks up all the cooking juices to become a delicious part of the meal.

¾ cup brown rice

1 cup halved cherry tomatoes

1 yellow bell pepper, diced

½ red onion, chopped

¼ cup sliced Kalamata olives

4 (4-ounce) boneless skinless chicken breasts, each cut into 3 pieces

2 teaspoons chopped fresh oregano

1 teaspoon garlic powder

2 cups sodium-free chicken stock or broth

Juice of ½ lemon

½ cup crumbled goat cheese

1 tablespoon chopped fresh parsley

1. Preheat the oven to 350ºF.

2. In a large bowl, stir together the brown rice, cherry tomatoes, yellow bell pepper, red onion, and olives. Spoon the mixture into a 9-by-13-inch baking dish.

3. Arrange the chicken breasts on top of the rice, and season them with oregano and garlic powder.

4. Pour the chicken stock and lemon juice over the chicken, vegetables, and rice.

5. Cover the dish and bake for 40 to 45 minutes, until the rice and chicken are cooked through.

6. Remove from the oven, uncover, and scatter the goat cheese and parsley over the casserole.

Substitution tip: Omit the chicken breasts and use vegetable stock to create a vegetarian meal. The goat cheese can stay unless a vegan designation is required.

PER SERVING Calories: 320; Total Fat: 11g; Saturated Fat: 4g; Carbohydrates: 29g; Fiber: 5g; Protein: 29g

Chicken Shepherd's Pie

SERVES 8 / PREP TIME: 20 MINUTES / COOK TIME: 50 MINUTES

Have you ever made mashed potatoes and ended up with a gluey mess rather than light, fluffy potatoes? Certain potatoes, such as russets, work better for mashing than others because they have a high starch content, which means the potato absorbs liquid easily and falls apart readily when mashed. For the best results stay away from white potatoes, red potatoes, and Yukon golds.

3 large russet potatoes, peeled and cut into 2-inch chunks

Sea salt

Freshly ground black pepper

1 tablespoon extra-virgin olive oil

1 sweet onion, peeled and chopped

1 tablespoon minced garlic

1 tablespoon cornstarch

2 cups sodium-free chicken stock or broth

1 teaspoon chopped fresh thyme

3 (5-ounce) boneless skinless chicken breasts, poached and cut into 1-inch chunks

2 carrots, peeled, cut into thin disks, and blanched

1½ cups peas

¼ cup grated Parmesan cheese

1. Preheat the oven to 325°F.

2. Fill a saucepan with cold water, place it over high heat, add the potatoes, and bring to a boil. Cook for about 20 minutes until soft.

3. Drain the potatoes, mash them, and season them with sea salt and pepper. Set aside.

4. While the potatoes cook, in a large skillet over medium-high heat, heat the olive oil.

5. Add the onion and garlic, and sauté for about 3 minutes until softened.

6. Whisk the cornstarch into the skillet to form a paste, and then whisk in the chicken stock until the sauce thickens.

7. Whisk in the thyme and season with sea salt and pepper.

8. Stir in the chicken, carrots, and peas. Spoon the chicken mixture into a 9-by-13-inch baking dish.

9. Spread the mashed potatoes over the top.

10. Sprinkle the potatoes with Parmesan cheese and bake for about 30 minutes until lightly browned.

Substitution tip: Mashed sweet potatoes can replace regular mashed for a colorful and tasty casserole. Prepare the sweet potatoes following the same instructions for preparing the russets.

PER SERVING Calories: 252; Total Fat: 6g; Saturated Fat: 2g; Carbohydrates: 29g; Fiber: 5g; Protein: 21g

Simple Chicken Cacciatore

SERVES 4 / PREP TIME: 20 MINUTES / COOK TIME: 35 MINUTES

Chicken cacciatore is often made with chicken thighs and braised in the oven for hours to create an intense tomato taste. This version uses chicken breast chunks and takes a shortcut to save cooking time. Sun-dried tomatoes add the concentrated tomato taste without the long cooking time. A tablespoon of tomato paste can also work well if sun-dried tomatoes are not available.

- 2 tablespoons extra-virgin olive oil
- 4 (4-ounce) boneless skinless chicken breasts, cut into 1-inch chunks
- 1 sweet onion, peeled and chopped
- 2 teaspoons minced garlic
- 2 celery stalks, chopped
- 1 large carrot, peeled and diced
- 1 red bell pepper, chopped
- 1 (15-ounce) can sodium-free diced tomatoes
- 1 cup quartered canned water-packed artichoke hearts
- ½ cup chopped sun-dried tomatoes
- 2 tablespoons chopped fresh oregano
- 2 tablespoons chopped fresh basil
- ½ teaspoon red pepper flakes
- Sea salt
- Freshly ground black pepper

1. In a large skillet over medium-high heat, heat the olive oil.
2. Add the chicken and cook for about 6 minutes, browning it on all sides.

3. Add the onion and garlic, and sauté for about 3 minutes until softened.

4. Stir in the celery, carrot, red bell pepper, tomatoes, artichoke hearts, sun-dried tomatoes, oregano, basil, and red pepper flakes. Cover and bring to a boil. Reduce the heat to low and simmer for about 25 minutes until the chicken is tender.

5. Season with sea salt and pepper.

6. Serve over rice or pasta, if desired.

Ingredient tip: Sun-drying tomatoes and other vegetables was a time-honored tradition to preserve delicate produce for winter or spring. Sun-dried tomatoes have a sweet taste and are packed with iron, potassium, copper, phosphorus, and manganese.

PER SERVING Calories: 355; Total Fat: 16g; Saturated Fat: 3g; Carbohydrates: 17g; Fiber: 6g; Protein: 36g

Spinach-Feta Chicken Burgers

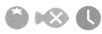

Imagine a balmy summer day spent with family and friends winding down on a shaded patio for a casual dinner. Hamburgers are a natural choice for such a meal and easy to prepare. Chicken burgers can be topped with the same condiments as regular beef burgers, and if you have a barbecue, fire it up and serve the burgers right off the grill.

1 pound lean ground chicken

1 large egg

1 scallion, white and green parts, chopped

½ cup finely chopped fresh spinach

½ cup homemade bread crumbs

¼ cup chopped sun-dried tomatoes

¼ cup crumbled feta cheese

1 teaspoon chopped fresh oregano

½ teaspoon minced garlic

1. Preheat the oven to 400°F.
2. In a large bowl, mix the chicken, egg, scallion, spinach, bread crumbs, sun-dried tomatoes, feta, oregano, and garlic. Form the chicken mixture into 4 equal patties and place them on a baking sheet. Bake for about 20 minutes, turning once, until cooked through.
3. Serve with a salad or on a bun with your favorite toppings.

Ingredient tip: Homemade bread crumbs are simple to make from stale bread, but you can also buy them at the grocery store for convenience. Most bakery sections have bags of store-made crumbs that contain no added sodium or preservatives.

PER SERVING Calories: 238; Total Fat: 9g; Saturated Fat: 4g; Carbohydrates: 11g; Fiber: 2g; Protein: 28g

Savory Turkey Meatballs

SERVES 4 / PREP TIME: 15 MINUTES / COOK TIME: 12 MINUTES

These unassuming minced meat creations are common world-wide. Delightfully versatile, they can be a tasty snack, added to your favorite sauce, or tucked into a sandwich for a hearty lunch. Lean ground pork or chicken can be used instead of turkey, or in combination for a taste variation.

1 pound lean ground turkey

1 large egg

½ sweet onion, peeled and finely diced

½ cup almond flour

2 teaspoons minced garlic

1 teaspoon chopped fresh basil

1 teaspoon chopped fresh thyme

Pinch sea salt

Pinch freshly ground black pepper

1. Preheat the oven to 350ºF.

2. Line a rimmed baking sheet with parchment paper and set aside.

3. In a large bowl, thoroughly mix the turkey, egg, onion, almond flour, garlic, basil, thyme, sea salt, and pepper.

4. Roll the turkey mixture into 1-inch meatballs and place them on the prepared sheet.

5. Bake the meatballs for about 12 minutes until they are browned and cooked through.

6. Serve with your favorite sauce or in a sandwich.

Ingredient tip: *To make almond flour at home, process blanched almonds in a food processor until ground. Just don't grind the nuts in the processor too long or you will end up with almond butter instead.*

PER SERVING Calories: 257; Total Fat: 15g; Saturated Fat: 3g; Carbohydrates: 5g; Fiber: 2g; Protein: 27g

Roasted Turkey Breast
with Herbs and Garlic

SERVES 4 / PREP TIME: 5 MINUTES / COOK TIME: 50 MINUTES

Chicken often overshadows turkey for everyday meals because the bigger bird is associated with massive dinners created for holidays or family events. Turkey is naturally higher in sodium than chicken but has fewer calories and contains no saturated fat. If you want your roast turkey to be very juicy, get a breast with the skin on, apply the rub underneath the skin, and then remove the skin after the meat is cooked.

2 tablespoons extra-
  virgin olive oil

2 teaspoons minced garlic

1 teaspoon chopped fresh thyme

½ teaspoon chopped
  fresh rosemary

½ teaspoon sea salt

½ teaspoon freshly
  ground black pepper

1½ pounds boneless
  skinless turkey breast

1. Preheat the oven to 350°F.

2. In a small bowl, stir together the olive oil, garlic, thyme, rosemary, sea salt, and pepper to form a rub.

3. Pat the turkey breast dry with paper towels.

4. Rub the garlic-herb mixture over the turkey breast and place it on a rimmed baking sheet.

5. Roast the turkey for about 50 minutes, or until a meat thermometer inserted into the thickest part of the breast reaches 165°F.

6. Remove the turkey from the oven, and let it rest for 10 minutes before serving.

Cooking tip: *Roast 2 turkey breasts, or a larger one, so you have lots of cooked meat leftover for other recipes or hearty sandwiches for lunch the next day. Just adjust the cooking time to ensure the meat is cooked through.*

PER SERVING Calories: 241; Total Fat: 10g; Saturated Fat: 2g; Carbohydrates: 8g; Fiber: 1g; Protein: 29g

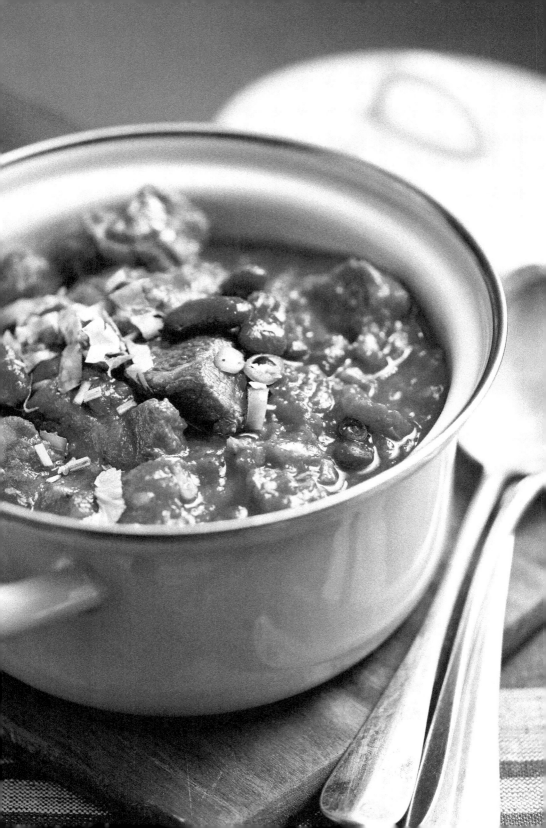

CHAPTER 11

Meat

Pork Chops with Fennel and Peaches

SERVES 4 / PREP TIME: 10 MINUTES / COOK TIME: 35 MINUTES

Pork is an often overlooked meat because people adopting healthier lifestyles gravitate toward chicken, fish, or vegetarian cuisine. Although it is a red meat, lean cuts, such as chops and tenderloin, are lower in calories and total fat than even the leanest cut of beef. Skinless chicken breast is higher in calories than pork.

2 tablespoons extra-virgin olive oil, divided, plus more for greasing the dish

4 (5-ounce) boneless pork chops, trimmed of visible fat

Sea salt

Freshly ground black pepper

½ fennel bulb, cut into 1-inch chunks

2 peaches, pitted and quartered

1 sweet onion, peeled and thinly sliced

2 tablespoons balsamic vinegar

1 teaspoon chopped fresh thyme

1. Preheat the oven to 400°F.

2. Lightly grease a 9-by-13-inch baking dish with olive oil and set aside.

3. Season the pork chops with sea salt and pepper.

4. In a large bowl, toss together the fennel, peaches, onion, balsamic vinegar, thyme, and 1 tablespoon of olive oil. Transfer the vegetables to the prepared dish and roast for 20 minutes.

5. In a large skillet over medium-high heat, heat the remaining 1 tablespoon of olive oil.

6. Add the chops and pan sear for about 2 minutes per side.

7. Remove the vegetables from the oven, stir them, and lay the pork chops on top.

8. Return the dish to the oven, and roast the meat and vegetables for about 10 minutes until the pork is just cooked through.

Cooking tip: *If you have a grill, cook the vegetables there in a foil packet, opening once to stir, and then simply grill the pork chops until the desired doneness. Serve them together on a large platter.*

PER SERVING Calories: 307; Total Fat: 12g; Saturated Fat: 3g; Carbohydrates: 10g; Fiber: 2g; Protein: 38g

Mediterranean Stuffed Pork Chops

SERVES 4 / PREP TIME: 15 MINUTES / COOK TIME: 20 MINUTES

The deep green flecks of basil and parsley in the slightly pink goat cheese filling look absolutely enchanting. Basil is not just a tasty, fragrant addition to recipes, though. It is also high in vitamin K, flavonoids, copper, and manganese. If you want to make the filling a couple days ahead, the antibacterial properties of this herb's essential oils will inhibit any bacterial growth.

¾ cup goat cheese

1 roasted red bell pepper, diced

1 tablespoon chopped fresh basil

1 tablespoon chopped fresh parsley

½ teaspoon minced garlic

4 (4-ounce) boneless pork chops, pounded to ¼-inch thickness

Sea salt

Freshly ground black pepper

2 tablespoons extra-virgin olive oil

½ cup sodium-free chicken stock or broth

1. In a small bowl, stir together the goat cheese, roasted red bell pepper, basil, parsley, and garlic.

2. Lay the pork chops on a cutting board and evenly divide the filling among the chops.

3. Fold the sides of the pork chops in and roll them to form a sealed package. Secure the pork closed with toothpicks. Lightly season on all sides with sea salt and pepper.

4. In a large skillet over medium-high heat, heat the olive oil.

5. Add the pork and cook for about 8 minutes, browning on all sides.

6. Add the chicken stock to the skillet, cover, and cook for about 10 minutes more, or until the pork is cooked through.

7. Remove and discard the toothpicks and serve.

Substitution tip: Chicken would taste delightful with this filling. Just pound the chicken breasts and assemble the dish the same way called for in the recipe. The only change would be increasing the cook time by at least 5 minutes.

PER SERVING Calories: 330; Total Fat: 19g; Saturated Fat: 8g; Carbohydrates: 3g; Fiber: 1g; Protein: 37g

Pork Chops with Wild Mushrooms

SERVES 4 / PREP TIME: 10 MINUTES / COOK TIME: 25 MINUTES

Mushrooms are earthy, sweet, and come in many wonderful varieties to enjoy. They are also the only vegetable that contains vitamin D, which means you should eat them during months that have limited natural sunshine. Mushrooms also help fight diseases, such as arthritis, cancer, and cardiovascular disease, while supporting the immune system. Try portobello, shiitake, oyster, enoki, and cremini mushrooms with the pork in this filling main course.

4 (5-ounce) bone-in center-
  cut pork chops

¼ teaspoon sea salt

¼ teaspoon freshly
  ground black pepper

1 tablespoon extra-virgin olive oil

1 sweet onion, chopped

2 teaspoons minced garlic

1 pound sliced mixed
  wild mushrooms

1 teaspoon chopped fresh thyme

½ cup sodium-free chicken
  stock or broth

1. Pat the pork chops dry with paper towels and season them with sea salt and pepper.

2. In a large skillet over medium-high heat, heat the olive oil.

3. Add the pork chops and cook for about 6 minutes, browning them on both sides. Transfer the meat to a plate and set aside.

4. In the same skillet, sauté the onion and garlic for about 3 minutes until softened.

5. Stir in the mushrooms and thyme and sauté for about 6 minutes more until the mushrooms are lightly caramelized and tender.

6. Return the pork chops to the skillet and pour in the chicken stock. Cover and bring the liquid to a boil. Reduce the heat to low and simmer for about 10 minutes until the chops are cooked through.

Cooking tip: *If you like your pork a little pink in the center, cut the cooking time here by about 4 minutes. There is no risk of trichinosis, which formerly was the reason for overcooking pork.*

PER SERVING Calories: 308; Total Fat: 17g; Saturated Fat: 5g; Carbohydrates: 7g; Fiber: 2g; Protein: 33g

Herb-Rubbed Pork Tenderloin

SERVES 8 / PREP TIME: 10 MINUTES / COOK TIME: 30 MINUTES

Herb rubs are a simple, low-calorie method of imparting taste to meats naturally mild in flavor. One of the stronger herbs you can use is rosemary, so a little goes a long way. Rosemary has stiff needles, which need to be stripped off the center stem and chopped very finely. This pungent herb is high in calcium, iron, and vitamins A and C, so eating it can reduce arthritis-related pain and help detoxify the liver.

¼ cup extra-virgin olive oil, plus 1 tablespoon

¼ cup chopped fresh oregano

¼ cup fresh chopped parsley

1 tablespoon finely chopped fresh rosemary

2 teaspoons minced garlic

½ teaspoon red pepper flakes

½ teaspoon sea salt

½ teaspoon freshly ground black pepper

2 pounds pork tenderloin, trimmed of visible fat and silver skin

1. Preheat the oven to 400°F.

2. In a food processor, process the ¼ cup of olive oil, the oregano, parsley, rosemary, garlic, red pepper flakes, sea salt, and pepper until a thick paste forms, scraping down the sides of the bowl at least once. Rub the herb mixture all over the pork tenderloin.

3. In a medium ovenproof skillet over medium-high heat, heat the remaining 1 tablespoon of olive oil.

4. Add the pork and sear the tenderloin on all sides, turning every 3 minutes until the meat is evenly browned.

5. Place the skillet in the oven and roast the tenderloin for about 20 minutes, or to the desired doneness. The internal temperature should be between 120ºF and 145ºF when measured with a meat thermometer.

6. Remove from the oven and let rest for 10 minutes before slicing and serving.

Ingredient tip: *Be careful when chopping parsley because it bruises very easily. Use a very sharp knife when preparing this herb. Bruised parsley will taste and smell like moldy grass after one day.*

PER SERVING Calories: 227; Total Fat: 10g; Saturated Fat: 2g; Carbohydrates: 2g; Fiber: 1g; Protein: 30g

Lamb Chops with Black Olive Pesto

SERVES 4 / PREP TIME: 10 MINUTES / COOK TIME: 25 MINUTES

Kalamata olives are a large, full-flavored, almost purple fruit often considered to be the best olive variety by chefs and foodies. Other black olives would work for this pesto, but the flavor might not be as distinctive. Olives are a fabulous source of vitamin E, iron, and fiber so they can help support heart health and boost the immune system.

For the pesto

½ cup pitted Kalamata olives

2 tablespoons chopped fresh parsley

2 tablespoons freshly squeezed lemon juice

1 tablespoon extra-virgin olive oil

2 teaspoons minced garlic

For the lamb chops

2 (½-pound) racks French-cut lamb chops

Sea salt

Freshly ground black pepper

1 tablespoon extra-virgin olive oil

To make the pesto

In a blender, pulse together the olives, parsley, lemon juice, olive oil, and garlic until the mixture is blended but still a little chunky. Set aside.

To make lamb chops

1. Preheat the oven to 450ºF.

2. Season the lamb with sea salt and pepper.

3. In a large ovenproof skillet over medium-high heat, heat the olive oil.

4. Add the lamb racks and pan sear for about 5 minutes, browning both sides and the bottom.

5. Arrange the racks, bone-side down, in the skillet and place it in the oven. Roast the lamb for about 20 minutes, or until the desired doneness. For medium-rare, the internal temperature should be 125ºF when measured with a meat thermometer.

6. Remove from the oven and let rest for 10 minutes. Cut the racks into chops, about 8 per rack.

7. Serve 4 chops per person and top with a spoonful of pesto.

Ingredient tip: *Olives should always be firm, with no dents or soft spots. If you like to buy olives from open olive bars in the super-market, make sure you add enough briny liquid to cover the fruit completely. You can keep these hand-selected olives only for about 2 weeks in the refrigerator. If you want to store them longer, buy product packed in jars.*

PER SERVING Calories: 295; Total Fat: 17g; Saturated Fat: 4g; Carbohydrates: 2g; Fiber: 1g; Protein: 32g

Broiled Flank Steak with Citrus Marinade

SERVES 4 / PREP TIME: 5 MINS, PLUS 30 MINS MARINATING / COOK TIME: 10 MINS

Orange juice plays three roles in this marinade: tenderizing, flavoring, and coloring. The acid in the juice helps break the protein bonds in the meat, as long as you don't marinate the steak for too long. A delicate orange flavor can still be detected after the flank steak is cooked and the natural sugars in the juice caramelize when exposed to heat. You can also grill the steak instead of broiling it.

¼ cup freshly squeezed orange juice

Juice of 1 lime

2 teaspoons minced garlic

2 teaspoon grated peeled fresh ginger

1 tablespoon chopped fresh cilantro

Pinch sea salt

Pinch freshly ground black pepper

1½ pounds flank steak

1. In a sealable plastic bag, combine the orange juice, lime juice, garlic, ginger, cilantro, sea salt, and pepper.

2. Add the steak, press out any excess air, and seal the bag. Refrigerate the steak for 30 minutes to marinate.

3. Preheat the oven to broil.

4. Remove the steak from the marinade and place it in a roasting dish with a rack.

5. Broil the steak for 5 minute per side for medium doneness.

6. Let the steak rest for 10 minutes before slicing it thinly across the grain.

Substitution tip: *More expensive cuts of beef, such as sirloin, can be used instead of flank steak but you will need to reduce the marinating time to about 15 minutes. Flank steak is a tougher cut, but has more flavor than tenderloin.*

PER SERVING Calories: 342; Total Fat: 14g; Saturated Fat: 6g; Carbohydrates: 3g; Fiber: 1g; Protein: 47g

Beef Sirloin Chili

SERVES 6 / PREP TIME: 15 MINUTES / COOK TIME: 1 HOUR

Cumin, used in this chili, is a spice used both in cooking and medicinally for centuries because it is packed with iron, magnesium, and calcium. Ancient healers administered cumin orally to boost the immune system and promote healthy digestion.

1 tablespoon extra-virgin olive oil

1 pound beef sirloin, cut into 1-inch chunks

1 sweet onion, peeled and chopped

1 red bell pepper, diced

2 teaspoons minced garlic

¼ cup chili powder

2 teaspoons ground cumin

1 teaspoon ground coriander

Pinch cayenne pepper

1 (28-ounce) can sodium-free diced tomatoes

1 (15-ounce) can dark red kidney beans, drained and rinsed

1 (15-ounce) can sodium-free white navy beans, drained and rinsed

2 tablespoons chopped scallion, green and white parts

2 tablespoons chopped cilantro (optional)

1. In a large saucepan over medium-high heat, heat the olive oil.

2. Add the beef and cook for about 10 minutes, browning it on all sides. Transfer the beef with a slotted spoon to a plate and set aside.

3. In the same pan, sauté the onion, red bell pepper, and garlic for about 3 minutes until softened.

4. Stir in the chili powder, cumin, coriander, cayenne pepper, tomatoes, kidney beans, white beans, and the reserved beef with any accumulated juices. Bring the chili to a boil and then reduce the heat to low. Simmer for about 50 minutes, or until the beef is tender.

5. Serve topped with scallion and cilantro, if using.

Substitution tip: *Dried beans can be soaked and cooked instead of using canned products in this chili. Canned beans are more convenient and health-conscious manufacturers offer many organic or sodium-free products.*

PER SERVING Calories: 347; Total Fat: 9g; Saturated Fat: 2g; Carbohydrates: 38g; Fiber: 11g; Protein: 34g

Beef Sirloin Veggie Kebabs

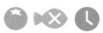

SERVES 4 / PREP TIME: 10 MINS, PLUS UP TO 6 HOURS MARINATING / COOK TIME: 10 MINS

You might feel like you are dining in a colorful bazaar when handed a plate of exotic looking kebabs for dinner. Zucchini adds color to the skewer, so it is important to buy firm, young squash that won't fall off when cooked. Zucchini is very high in vitamins A and C, fiber, manganese, and copper. Either yellow squash or zucchini, or both, will work in this dish.

2 tablespoons extra-virgin olive oil

2 tablespoons balsamic vinegar

2 teaspoons minced garlic

1 teaspoon chopped fresh rosemary

1 teaspoon chopped fresh thyme

½ teaspoon freshly ground black pepper

1 pound top sirloin steak, trimmed of visible fat, and cut into 2-inch chunks

1 red onion, peeled, quartered, and separated into layers

1 red bell pepper, seeded and cut into 1½-inch chunks (about 8)

1 zucchini, cut into 1½-inch chunks (about 8)

1. In a medium bowl, stir together the olive oil, balsamic vinegar, garlic, rosemary, thyme, and pepper until well blended.

2. Add the beef chunks and stir to coat. Cover the bowl and refrigerate for up to 6 hours to marinate, stirring occasionally.

3. Preheat the oven to broil.

4. Assemble the kebabs alternating pieces of beef with red onion, red bell pepper, and zucchini. Place the finished kebabs on a roasting rack.

5. Broil the kebabs for about 10 minutes for medium, turning once or twice, until the beef is cooked to your desired doneness.

6. Transfer the kebabs to a plate and let them rest for 5 minutes before serving.

Cooking tip: *Kebabs can be cooked easily on a medium-high grill if weather permits. Soak wooden skewers well in water before threading on the meat and vegetables.*

PER SERVING Calories: 305; Total Fat: 14g; Saturated Fat: 4g; Carbohydrates: 7g; Fiber: 2g; Protein: 36g

Sun-Dried Tomato Meatloaf

SERVES 4 / PREP TIME: 10 MINUTES / COOK TIME: 50 MINUTES

Humble meatloaf has been transformed from a dish served in diners to haute cuisine. Fresh basil and sun-dried tomatoes elevate this recipe to somewhere in between. You might want to double the recipe because nothing beats cold meatloaf on a crusty multigrain bun for lunch.

1 pound lean ground beef (92%)

½ sweet onion, chopped

1 large egg

½ cup homemade bread crumbs

¼ cup chopped sun-dried tomatoes

¼ cup milk

2 tablespoons chopped fresh basil

1 teaspoon minced garlic

1 teaspoon chopped fresh parsley

Pinch sea salt

Pinch freshly ground black pepper

Pinch red pepper flakes

1. Preheat the oven to 350°F.

2. In a large bowl, thoroughly mix the ground beef, onion, egg, bread crumbs, sun-dried tomatoes, milk, basil, garlic, parsley, sea salt, pepper, and red pepper flakes.

3. Press the meatloaf mixture into a 9-by-5-inch loaf pan and bake for about 50 minutes until the meatloaf is cooked through.

4. Remove from the oven and let stand for 10 minutes. Pour out any accumulated grease, slice, and serve.

Substitution tip: Use lean ground pork or venison for a different taste profile when you want to experiment. But keep the amount of meat you use to one pound, so the texture does not suffer.

PER SERVING Calories: 305; Total Fat: 10g; Saturated Fat: 3g; Carbohydrates: 14g; Fiber: 1g; Protein: 39g

Beef Patties (Kefta)

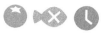

Kefta is the Moroccan word for "ground meat," particularly ground beef, lamb, or a combination, and is a popular dish found in Middle Eastern and central and south Asian cuisines. Kefta can be compared to the American meatball or meatloaf dishes.

1 pound lean ground beef (92%)

½ cup chopped fresh parsley

1 sweet onion, diced

2 garlic cloves, minced

1 tablespoon allspice

1½ teaspoons sea salt

¼ teaspoon freshly ground black pepper

¼ teaspoon ground cinnamon

¼ teaspoon ground cumin

1. Preheat the boiler to high.

2. Line a baking sheet with aluminum foil and set a wire rack on it. Set aside.

3. In a food processor, pulse together the ground beef, parsley, onion, garlic, allspice, sea salt, pepper, cinnamon, and cumin until coarsely mixed.

4. Using about 3 tablespoons of the meat mixture for each, form 4 to 6 thin patties. Place them on the wire rack.

5. Broil the patties for 3 minutes, flip, and cook for 2 to 3 minutes more, testing after 2 minutes. They should be browned and cooked through.

Preparation tip: Gently shape the meat mixture into slightly oval-shaped burgers. Using two fingers, make a small indention in the center of each burger to prevent swelling while cooking.

PER SERVING Calories: 152; Total Fat: 5g; Saturated Fat: 2g; Carbohydrates: 3g; Fiber: 1g; Protein: 23g

Beef Stifado

SERVES 6 / PREP TIME: 15 MINUTES / COOK TIME: 1 HOUR, 45 MINUTES

Stifado is basically an onion and beef stew flavored with red wine, vinegar, and cinnamon. Any type of stewing beef will work here, but you want a cut with lots of connective tissue (collagen), which melts as the meat cooks, creating a succulent flavor. This stew freezes beautifully, so package up any leftovers and store them for another delicious meal.

1 tablespoon extra-virgin olive oil

2 pounds chuck steak, trimmed of fat and cut into thin strips

2 sweet onions, peeled and diced

2 teaspoons minced garlic

1 (28-ounce) can sodium-free diced tomatoes with juice

¼ cup dry red wine

1 tablespoon balsamic vinegar

2 dried bay leaves

1 teaspoon dried oregano

½ teaspoon ground cinnamon

Dash ground allspice

Sea salt

Freshly ground black pepper

1. Preheat the oven to 350°F.

2. In a large ovenproof skillet over medium-high heat, heat the olive oil.

3. Brown the beef in batches, transferring it to a plate when finished. Cook time is about 10 minutes total.

4. Add the onions and garlic, and sauté for about 3 minutes until softened.

5. Stir in the tomatoes, red wine, balsamic vinegar, bay leaves, oregano, cinnamon, allspice, and the reserved beef with any accumulated juices. Cover the skillet and put it into the oven. Roast for about 1½ hours until the meat is very tender, stirring occasionally.

6. Remove and discard the bay leaves. Season with sea salt and pepper, and serve.

Cooking tip: The alcohol in the red wine cooks off as the stew simmers, so the dish is still appropriate for minors or those who cannot drink alcohol.

PER SERVING Calories: 319; Total Fat: 18g; Saturated Fat: 1g; Carbohydrates: 8g; Fiber: 2g; Protein: 33g

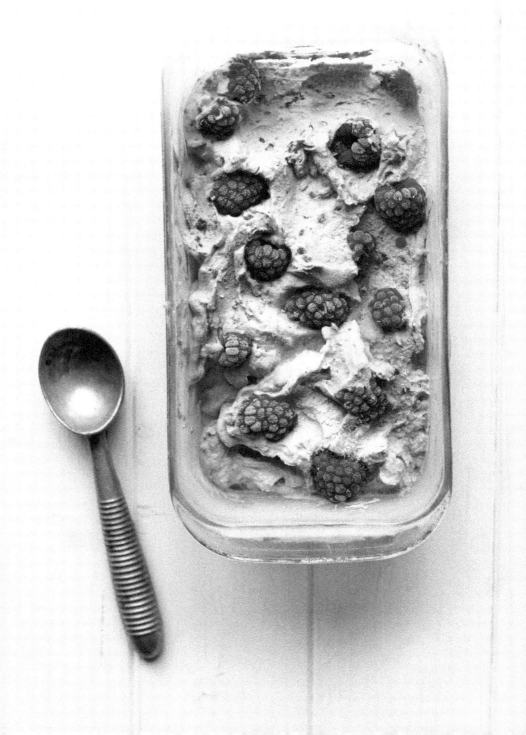

CHAPTER 12

Desserts

Honey Panna Cotta

SERVES 6 / PREP TIME: 10 MINUTES, PLUS 4 HOURS OR OVERNIGHT CHILLING /
COOK TIME: 5 MINUTES

Gelatin might not be an ingredient you use very often, but don't let that scare you away from this luscious dessert. You need the gelatin to create the signature texture of the panna cotta, and it is important to follow a few important steps for success. Never boil the gelatin or it will not set. Use the gelatin mixture right after it is hydrated or you might end up with a solid inedible mass. Either gelatin sheets or granules will work fine for this recipe.

4 teaspoons unflavored gelatin

3 cups heavy (whipping) cream

6 tablespoons honey

1 teaspoon pure vanilla extract

½ teaspoon almond extract

1. In a small bowl, stir together the gelatin and ½ cup of heavy cream. Set aside to soften.

2. In a medium saucepan over medium-high heat, heat the remaining 2½ cups of heavy cream until just below boiling. Remove the pan from the heat.

3. Whisk in the honey, vanilla extract, and almond extract, whisking for about 3 minutes until the honey dissolves.

4. Whisk in the gelatin mixture and pour the panna cotta into a 4-cup serving dish.

5. Place the dish in the refrigerator for at least 4 hours, or overnight, to set.

6. Carefully run a knife around the edge of the panna cotta. Place a serving plate over the dish and carefully invert the dish to release the pudding.

7. Serve.

Substitution tip: Gelatin is an animal-based gelling agent, so vegetarians and vegans cannot use it. If you prefer a vegetarian dessert, try the seaweed-based carrageen or agar-agar instead of gelatin.

PER SERVING Calories: 274; Total Fat: 22g; Saturated Fat: 14g; Carbohydrates: 19g; Fiber: 17g; Protein: 1g

Raspberry Frozen Yogurt

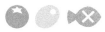

SERVES 4 / PREP TIME: 25 MINUTES, PLUS FREEZING AND SCRAPING DOWN TIME

You do not need an ice-cream maker to make this creamy pink dessert, but it does help create a smooth, easy-to-spoon texture. If a soft-serve style frozen treat is preferred, transfer the frozen yogurt to a food processor just before serving and pulse until all the frozen chunks are puréed. You can refreeze any leftovers.

4 cups fresh raspberries

1 cup plain Greek yogurt

¼ cup honey

1 tablespoon freshly squeezed lemon juice

1. In a food processor, place 3 cups of the raspberries, yogurt, honey, and lemon juice and pulse until mixed.
2. Pass the mixture through a fine-mesh sieve.
3. Stir in remaining 1 cup raspberries into yogurt mixture.
4. Pour the raspberry yogurt into a metal baking dish and freeze until the edges are solid.
5. Stir, scraping the hardened bits from the side and return to the freezer. Freeze until the edges are solid and scrape again. Repeat this process until the yogurt is completely frozen and serve.

Substitution tip: Any fruit would be delicious when blended with tangy yogurt, so throw in fresh blueberries, peaches, plums, strawberries, and even chunks of orange for a cool variation. Depending on the sweetness of your fruit, adjust the amount of honey or omit it completely.

PER SERVING Calories: 184; Total Fat: 4g; Saturated Fat: 2g; Carbohydrates: 36g; Fiber: 8g; Protein: 4g

Strawberry–Chia Seed Pudding

SERVES 4 / PREP TIME: 5 MINUTES, PLUS 4 HOURS OR OVERNIGHT CHILLING

*Chia seeds are entirely too healthy to be used for dessert—
they are a complete protein and higher in omega-3 fatty acids
than salmon. However, combined with creamy almond milk,
bright berries, and a touch of vanilla, chia seeds become a
decadent treat. Whenever possible, purchase organic seeds
because although they are gathered by hand, chia seeds can
have pesticide traces.*

2 cups unsweetened almond milk

¼ cup chia seeds

1 tablespoon pure vanilla extract

2 tablespoons honey

2 cups sliced fresh strawberries

1. In a medium bowl, stir together the almond milk, chia seeds, vanilla, and honey.

2. Place the bowl, covered, in the refrigerator for at least 4 hours, or overnight.

3. Serve the pudding topped with strawberries.

*Ingredient tip: For superior taste and quality, local strawberries in
season are the best choice for this recipe. These sweet beauties are
very perishable, so even a few days in the refrigerator can reduce vitamin C levels and leave you with berries that have soft spots or mold.*

PER SERVING Calories: 108; Total Fat: 4g; Saturated Fat: 0g; Carbohydrates: 18g; Fiber: 5g;
Protein: 3g

Fruit-Nut Crumble

SERVES 4 / PREP TIME: 20 MINUTES

Strawberries are just one of the fruits in this filling, but their sweetness and heady fragrance shines through in every bite. Strawberries are an excellent source of beta-carotene, vitamin C, potassium, ellagic acid, and iron. This berry can fight cancer, cut the risk of cardiovascular disease, improve the immune system, and stabilize blood sugar.

1 cup rolled oats

¼ cup pecan pieces

¼ cup hazelnuts

¼ cup pitted dates

¼ cup dried cranberries

½ teaspoon pure vanilla extract

½ teaspoon ground cinnamon

1 cup sliced fresh strawberries

2 kiwis, peeled and diced

1 peach, pitted and diced

1 plum, pitted and diced

½ cup fresh blueberries

1. In a food processor, pulse the oats, pecans, hazelnuts, dates, cranberries, vanilla extract, and cinnamon until crumbly and well mixed.

2. In a large bowl, toss together the strawberries, kiwis, peach, plum, and blueberries. Divide the fruit among four bowls.

3. Top each with equal amounts of the crumble and serve.

Ingredient tip: Kiwi is on the Environmental Working Group's Clean 15 list. This means kiwi is one of the least-contaminated-by-pesticide produce choices in the United States.

PER SERVING Calories: 228; Total Fat: 7g; Saturated Fat: 1g; Carbohydrates: 39g; Fiber: 7g; Protein: 5g

Fresh Gingered Melon

SERVES 4 / PREP TIME: 15 MINUTES

Desserts don't need to be elaborate or heavy to be satisfying. A few simple, incredibly fresh ingredients can be the best ending for a backyard barbecue or dinner enjoyed with friends or family. Throw in a little chopped mint for extra freshness and pretty contrasting color.

½ cantaloupe, peeled and cut into 1-inch chunks

2 cups 1-inch watermelon chunks

2 cups 1-inch honeydew melon chunks

2 tablespoons honey

Juice of 1 (2-inch) piece grated peeled fresh ginger

1. In a large bowl, place the cantaloupe, watermelon, and honeydew melon chunks.

2. Stir in the honey and ginger juice (usually about a couple drops) to combine and serve.

Ingredient tip: Picking a perfect watermelon can seem like an uncertain task because you really don't know what the melon will be like until you cut it open. To increase your chances of getting a ripe, firm watermelon, look for one that is deep green with a creamy yellowish spot on one side.

PER SERVING Calories: 91; Total Fat: 0g; Saturated Fat: 0g; Carbohydrates: 24g; Fiber: 1g; Protein: 1g

Quinoa Fruit Salad

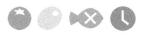

SERVES 4 / PREP TIME: 25 MINUTES

Mangos are one of the most succulent and glorious fruits, with silky flesh and an intoxicating, almost piney, fragrance. Mangos can also be one of the harder fruits to cut up and prepare due to its strange flat pit. Don't try to peel the mango first, because it will easily slip away when you cut around the pit. Instead, cut the flesh off each side of the pit and then remove the skin after.

2 tablespoons honey

2 tablespoons freshly
  squeezed lime juice

1 teaspoon chopped fresh basil

1 cup cooked quinoa

1 cup sliced fresh strawberries

1 cup fresh blackberries

1 mango, peeled, pitted, and diced

1 peach, pitted and diced

2 kiwis, peeled and quartered

1. In a small bowl, stir together the honey, lime juice, and basil. Set aside.

2. In a large bowl, stir together the quinoa, strawberries, blackberries, mango, peach, and kiwis.

3. Add the honey mixture to the fruit salad and toss to coat.

Cooking tip: Rinse quinoa in cold water before using it because you might be sensitive to the soapy coating, called saponin, found in each seed.

PER SERVING Calories: 206; Total Fat: 2g; Saturated Fat: 0g; Carbohydrates: 45g; Fiber: 7g; Protein: 5g

Stuffed Figs with Goat Cheese

SERVES 6 / PREP TIME: 10 MINUTES / COOK TIME: 10 MINUTES

One tree in particular and native to the Middle East, the fig tree, produces my favorite fruit. Besides being very nutritious, figs are exotic—their abundance of flavor, color, texture, and appearance are irresistible. Figs contain a lot of minerals, vitamins, antioxidants, and are high in dietary fiber.

10 fresh figs, halved

4 ounces goat cheese, divided

20 almonds, chopped

2 tablespoons honey

1. Preheat the broiler to high.
2. Place the fig halves, cut-side up, on a baking sheet.
3. Top each with about ½ teaspoon of goat cheese.
4. Sprinkle about 1 teaspoon of almonds on each fig.
5. Broil the figs for 2 to 3 minutes until the cheese is soft and the almonds have a nice golden color. Remove the figs from the oven and let cool for 5 minutes.
6. Drizzle the honey on top and serve warm.

Ingredient tip: Can't find fresh figs? No problem. Top your favorite salad with dried figs so you can still enjoy their health benefits.

PER SERVING Calories: 209; Total Fat: 9g; Saturated Fat: 5g; Carbohydrates: 27g; Fiber: 4g; Protein: 8g

Dessert Crêpes with Fresh Berries

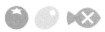

SERVES 4 / PREP TIME: 10 MINUTES, PLUS 2 HOURS RESTING / COOK TIME: 20 MINUTES

These days many people have some type of dairy or soy sensitivity, so almond milk stands in as a perfect alternative. Almond milk is also a popular choice for those with diabetes because it does not impact blood sugar and is very low in carbohydrates. You can use other nut milks, such as cashew or coconut, without affecting the texture or taste of these tender crêpes.

1¼ cups unsweetened almond milk

3 large eggs

¾ cup whole-wheat flour

½ cup all-purpose flour

¼ teaspoon sea salt

Extra-virgin olive oil, for cooking

4 cups mixed fresh berries

1. In medium bowl, whisk the milk and eggs until blended.

2. In another medium bowl, stir together the whole-wheat flour, all-purpose flour, and sea salt.

3. Add the dry ingredients to the wet ingredients and whisk until the batter is smooth. Set aside to rest for 2 hours.

4. Place a crêpe pan or small non-stick skillet over medium-high heat and brush a small amount of olive oil onto the bottom of the pan.

5. Pour ¼ cup of batter into the skillet and swirl the pan until the bottom is completely covered.

6. Cook the crêpe for 1 minute, flip, and cook the other side for 1 minute more until lightly browned. Transfer the cooked crêpe to a plate. Repeat the cooking process with the remaining batter.

7. Wrap the crêpes around the berries and serve 2 per person.

Cooking tip: *Crêpes freeze beautifully if packaged correctly, so double this recipe for an easy snack or breakfast later. Make the crêpes and place them between sheets of parchment paper so they can't stick together and then slide the whole stack into a large sealable freezer bag.*

PER SERVING Calories: 251; Total Fat: 5g; Saturated Fat: 1g; Carbohydrates: 41g; Fiber: 4g; Protein: 10g

Citrus Polenta

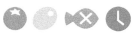

SERVES 4 / PREP TIME: 10 MINUTES / COOK TIME: 5 MINUTES

Polenta is a staple food in northern Italy and is similar to the grits served in the southern United States, but with a longer history. In ancient times, yeast and grain mills were difficult to access for most people, so this paste, made from grains and water, was common. Polenta is prized for its versatility and can be served as a savory dish or as a sweetened dessert, such as this one.

3 cups unsweetened almond milk	½ cup plain Greek yogurt
1 cup water	¼ cup honey, divided
¼ teaspoon sea salt	2 teaspoons orange zest, divided
1 cup fine cornmeal	1 teaspoon lemon zest, divided

1. In a large saucepan over medium-high heat, place the almond milk, water, and sea salt. Bring to a boil.

2. Slowly whisk in the cornmeal and return the mixture to a boil. Reduce the heat to low and simmer, whisking for about 3 minutes until the mixture thickens.

3. Remove the saucepan from the heat, cover, and let stand for 10 minutes to thicken further.

4. In a small bowl, stir together the yogurt, 1 tablespoon of honey, 1 teaspoon of orange zest, and ½ teaspoon of lemon zest. Set aside.

5. Whisk the remaining 3 tablespoons of honey, 1 teaspoon of orange zest, and ½ teaspoon of lemon zest into the polenta.

6. Spoon the polenta into 4 bowls and top each with a generous spoonful of the yogurt topping.

Ingredient tip: *If you don't purchase organic lemons, take the time to scrub the fruit extensively to remove the wax coating applied to protect the fruit during transport. You want to add lemon zest to the polenta, not wax.*

PER SERVING Calories: 224; Total Fat: 5g; Saturated Fat: 1g; Carbohydrates: 43g; Fiber: 6g; Protein: 4g

Spiced Pear and Applesauce

SERVES 4 / PREP TIME: 15 MINUTES / COOK TIME: 20 MINUTES

Pears are not a usual ingredient in applesauce, but they serve as a distinctive component in this variation. Almost any ingredient can be added to puréed apples with success, even carrots or berries, but pears seem to create a complexity of flavor pleasing to the palate. Leave the skin on the pears and apples if you wish, because that part of the fruit contains about half of the dietary fiber. The skin is also packed with antioxidants that can help fight disease.

4 pears, peeled, cored, and chopped

2 tart apples, peeled, cored, and chopped

¼ cup water

2 tablespoons honey

½ teaspoon ground cinnamon

¼ teaspoon ground nutmeg

Pinch ground cloves

1. In medium saucepan over medium heat, place the pears, apples, water, honey, cinnamon, nutmeg, and cloves. Cover and bring the mixture to a boil. Reduce the heat to low and cook the fruit for about 20 minutes until it is soft.

2. Remove the pot from the heat and mash the mixture until it is mostly smooth, but still a little chunky.

3. Cool and serve.

Cooking tip: If you want a very convenient method for preparing this dessert, try a slow cooker. Simply place all the ingredients in the cooker, set it to low, and cook until the desired texture is reached.

PER SERVING Calories: 202; Total Fat: 1g; Saturated Fat: 0g; Carbohydrates: 53g; Fiber: 9g; Protein: 1g

APPENDIX A: THE DIRTY DOZEN AND THE CLEAN FIFTEEN

A nonprofit and environmental watchdog organization called Environmental Working Group (EWG) looks at data supplied by the US Department of Agriculture (USDA) and the Food and Drug Administration (FDA) about pesticide residues and compiles a list each year of the best and worst pesticide loads found in commercial crops. You can refer to the Dirty Dozen list to know which fruits and vegetables you should always buy organic. The Clean Fifteen list lets you know which produce is considered safe enough when grown conventionally to allow you to skip the organics. This does not mean that the Clean Fifteen produce is pesticide-free, though, so wash these fruits and vegetables thoroughly.

These lists change every year, so make sure you look up the most recent before you fill your shopping cart. You'll find the most recent lists as well as a guide to pesticides in produce at EWG.org/FoodNews.

2016 Dirty Dozen

Apples	Nectarines	Sweet bell peppers	*with highly toxic organo-phosphate insecticides:*
Celery	Peaches		
Cherry tomatoes	Potatoes	*In addition to the Dirty Dozen, the EWG added two foods contaminated*	
Cucumbers	Snap peas		Hot peppers
Grapes	Spinach		Kale/Collard greens
	Strawberries		

2016 Clean Fifteen

Asparagus	Cauliflower	Mangoes	Sweet corn
Avocados	Eggplant	Onions	Sweet peas (frozen)
Cabbage	Grapefruit	Papayas	
Cantaloupe	Kiwis	Pineapples	Sweet potatoes

243

APPENDIX B: MEASUREMENT CONVERSIONS

Volume Equivalents (Liquid)

US STANDARD	US STANDARD (OUNCES)	METRIC (APPROXIMATE)
2 tablespoons	1 fl. oz.	30 mL
¼ cup	2 fl. oz.	60 mL
½ cup	4 fl. oz.	120 mL
1 cup	8 fl. oz.	240 mL
1½ cups	12 fl. oz.	355 mL
2 cups or 1 pint	16 fl. oz.	475 mL
4 cups or 1 quart	32 fl. oz.	1 L
1 gallon	128 fl. oz.	4 L

Oven Temperatures

FAHRENHEIT (F)	CELSIUS (C) (APPROXIMATE)
250°F	120°C
300°F	150°C
325°F	165°C
350°F	180°C
375°F	190°C
400°F	200°C
425°F	220°C
450°F	230°C

Volume Equivalents (Dry)

US STANDARD	METRIC (APPROXIMATE)
⅛ teaspoon	0.5 mL
¼ teaspoon	1 mL
½ teaspoon	2 mL
¾ teaspoon	4 mL
1 teaspoon	5 mL
1 tablespoon	15 mL
¼ cup	59 mL
⅓ cup	79 mL
½ cup	118 mL
⅔ cup	156 mL
¾ cup	177 mL
1 cup	235 mL
2 cups or 1 pint	475 mL
3 cups	700 mL
4 cups or 1 quart	1 L
½ gallon	2 L
1 gallon	4 L

Weight Equivalents

US STANDARD	METRIC (APPROXIMATE)
½ ounce	15 g
1 ounce	30 g
2 ounces	60 g
4 ounces	115 g
8 ounces	225 g
12 ounces	340 g
16 ounces or 1 pound	455 g

REFERENCES

Altomare, Roberta, Francesco Cacciabauda, Giuseppe Damiano, Vincenzo Davide Palumbo, Maria Concetta Gioviale, Maurizio Bellavia, Giovanni Tomasello, and Attilio Ignazio Lo Monte. "The Mediterranean Diet: A History of Health." *Iranian Journal of Public Health* 42, no. 5 (May 2013): 449–57. Accessed April 1, 2016. www.ncbi.nlm.nih.gov/pmc/articles/PMC3684452/.

American Heart Association. "Heart Disease and Stroke Statistics—2016 Update." Accessed April 1, 2016. circ.ahajournals.org/content/early /2015/12/16/CIR.0000000000000350.

American Heart Association. "Mediterranean Diet." Accessed April 3, 2016. www.heart.org/HEARTORG/HealthyLiving/HealthyEating/Mediterranean-Diet_UCM_306004_Article.jsp#.VzYn0YQrJD8.

American Stroke Association. "Heart Disease, Stroke, and Research Statistics At-a-Glance." Accessed April 2, 2016. www.heart.org/idc/groups/ahamah-public/@wcm/@sop/@smd/documents/downloadable/ucm_480086.pdf.

Berry, E. M., Y. Arnoni, and M. Aviram. "The Middle Eastern and Biblical Origins of the Mediterranean Diet." *Public Health Nutrition* 14, no. 12A (December 2011): 2288–95. Accessed April 2, 2016. doi:10.1017/S1368980011002539.

Crous-Bou, Marta, Teresa T. Fung, Jennifer Prescott, Bettina Julin, Mengmeng Du, Qi Sun, Kathryn M. Rexrode, et al. "Mediterranean Diet and Telomere Length in Nurses' Health Study: Population-Based Cohort Study." *British Medical Journal* 349 (December 2014). Accessed April 1, 2016. doi:http://dx.doi.org/10.1136/bmj.g6674.

Esposito K., C. M. Kastorini, D. B. Panagiotakos, and D. Giugliano. "Mediterranean Diet and Weight Loss: Meta-Analysis of Randomized Controlled Trials." *Metabolic Syndrome and Related Disorders* 9, no. 1 (February 2011): 1–12. doi:10.1089/met.2010.0031.

Epicurious. "The Mediterranean Diet." Accessed April 5, 2016. www.epicurious.com/archive/healthy/news/diet_mediterranean.

Estruch, Ramón, Emilio Ros, Jordi Salas-Salvadó, Maria-Isabel Covas, Dolores Corella, Fernando Arós, Enrique Gómez-Gracia, et al., "Primary Prevention of Cardiovascular Disease with a Mediterranean Diet." *New England Journal of Medicine* 368 (April 2013): 1279–90. Accessed April 2, 2016. doi:10.1056/NEJ Moa1200303.

Keys, Ancel, C. Aravanis, and H. Blackburn, eds. *The Seven Countries: A Multivariate Analysis of Death and Coronary Heart Disease*. Cambridge, MA: Harvard University Press, 1980.

Keys, Ancel, ed. "Coronary Heart Disease in Seven Countries." *Circulation* 41, Suppl. 1 (1970): 1–211.

National Heart, Lung, and Blood Institute. "Disease Statistics." Accessed April 2, 2016. www.nhlbi.nih.gov/about/documents/factbook/2012/chapter4.

Office of Disease and Prevention and Health Promotion. "Appendix 4. USDA Food Patterns: Healthy Mediterranean-Style Eating Pattern." *Dietary Guidelines for Americans 2015–2020*. 8 ed. Accessed April 1, 2016. http://health.gov/dietaryguidelines/2015/guidelines/appendix-4/.

Samieri, Cécilia, Qi Sun, Mary K. Townsend, Stephanie E. Chiuve, Olivia I. Okereke, Walter C. Willett, Meir Stampfer, and Francine Grodstein. "The Association between Dietary Patterns at Midlife and Health in Aging: An Observational Study." *Annals of Internal Medicine* 159, no. 9 (November 2013): 584–91. Accessed April 1, 2016. doi:10.7326/0003-4819-159-9-201311050-00004.

RECIPE INDEX

247

INDEX

ACKNOWLEDGMENTS

First and foremost, I have to thank my parents for their love and support. My upbringing in Lebanon is what brought this book to life. Thank you both for giving me the strength to reach for the stars and chase my dreams. My siblings—Marie, David, Abdo, and Tony deserve my wholehearted appreciation—you are my rocks.

Second, I would like to thank everyone who helped me complete this book—to all those who provided support, talked through my ideas, read, wrote, offered comments, assisted in the editing, proofreading, and design.

I would like to thank Michelle Anderson, Mary Cassells, Therezia Alchoufete, and Joyce Tielsch for helping me through the process of selecting recipes and editing drafts.

A warm thank-you to Meg Ilasco—once again, thank you so much for helping me make this happen.

ABOUT THE AUTHOR

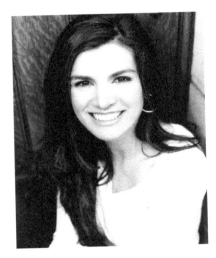

Susan Zogheib was born in Beirut, Lebanon, and moved to the United States with her family in the late 1980s. She is a registered dietitian (RD) and holds a master's degree from Ryerson University in Toronto, Ontario, in nutrition communication. Susan is a food and nutrition expert and media consultant with more than ten years' experience working as a clinical dietitian. You can find her online at susueats.com, @susueats on Instagram, and facebook.com/susueats. She currently lives in Pittsburgh, Pennsylvania.

Her philosophy on food and nutrition: She chooses foods that will nourish you—inside and out. Every body is different and you should make your food work for you. Quick fixes do not exist; it takes hard work and dedication to create and live a nutritious life.